HUMAN ANATOMY AND PHYSIOLOGY

ANTHROPOMETRY

TYPES, USES AND APPLICATIONS

HUMAN ANATOMY AND PHYSIOLOGY

Additional books and e-books in this series can be found on Nova's website under the Series tab.

HUMAN ANATOMY AND PHYSIOLOGY

ANTHROPOMETRY

TYPES, USES AND APPLICATIONS

SÉBASTIEN LEGRAND
EDITOR

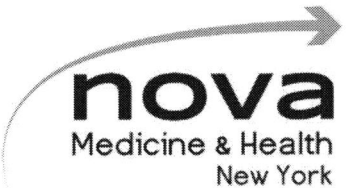

Copyright © 2021 by Nova Science Publishers, Inc.

All rights reserved. No part of this book may be reproduced, stored in a retrieval system or transmitted in any form or by any means: electronic, electrostatic, magnetic, tape, mechanical photocopying, recording or otherwise without the written permission of the Publisher.

We have partnered with Copyright Clearance Center to make it easy for you to obtain permissions to reuse content from this publication. Simply navigate to this publication's page on Nova's website and locate the "Get Permission" button below the title description. This button is linked directly to the title's permission page on copyright.com. Alternatively, you can visit copyright.com and search by title, ISBN, or ISSN.

For further questions about using the service on copyright.com, please contact:
Copyright Clearance Center
Phone: +1-(978) 750-8400   Fax: +1-(978) 750-4470   E-mail: info@copyright.com.

NOTICE TO THE READER

The Publisher has taken reasonable care in the preparation of this book, but makes no expressed or implied warranty of any kind and assumes no responsibility for any errors or omissions. No liability is assumed for incidental or consequential damages in connection with or arising out of information contained in this book. The Publisher shall not be liable for any special, consequential, or exemplary damages resulting, in whole or in part, from the readers' use of, or reliance upon, this material. Any parts of this book based on government reports are so indicated and copyright is claimed for those parts to the extent applicable to compilations of such works.

Independent verification should be sought for any data, advice or recommendations contained in this book. In addition, no responsibility is assumed by the Publisher for any injury and/or damage to persons or property arising from any methods, products, instructions, ideas or otherwise contained in this publication.

This publication is designed to provide accurate and authoritative information with regard to the subject matter covered herein. It is sold with the clear understanding that the Publisher is not engaged in rendering legal or any other professional services. If legal or any other expert assistance is required, the services of a competent person should be sought. FROM A DECLARATION OF PARTICIPANTS JOINTLY ADOPTED BY A COMMITTEE OF THE AMERICAN BAR ASSOCIATION AND A COMMITTEE OF PUBLISHERS.

Additional color graphics may be available in the e-book version of this book.

Library of Congress Cataloging-in-Publication Data

ISBN: 978-1-53619-269-8

Published by Nova Science Publishers, Inc. † New York

CONTENTS

Preface		vii
Chapter 1	Association between Novel Anthropometric Parameters and Cardiovascular Risk Factors among Obese Adults *Wattana Leowattana*	1
Chapter 2	Anthropometry of Children Age 0-12 Years, in the Senegal River Valley in 1957: Situation and Perspectives *Michel Garenne and Pierre Cantrelle*	39
Chapter 3	Obesity and Anthropometry *Archana Khanna*	75
Chapter 4	The Effect of Different Types of Exercise on Anthropometric Measures and Body Composition in Older Adults *Pablo Monteagudo*	95
Index		115

PREFACE

In Anthropometry: Types, Uses and Applications, the science of anthropometry, which deals with measurements of human size, shape and proportion, is examined in the context of obesity and overweight, common problems in developed countries and developing countries alike. An estimated 39% of the world's adult population were overweight and 13% were obese over the past 3 decades, and these problems can cause diseases like type 2 diabetes mellitus (T2DM), cardiovascular diseases (CVD), and several cancers. While body mass index (BMI) is commonly used as a health risk phenotype, it has several limitations because BMI does not accurately depict different components of body composition and is therefore unable to predict the prognostic effect of individual tissues. Other anthropometric measurements, such as waist circumference (WC), waist to hip ratio (WHR), and waist to height ratio (WHtR) each have their advantages and disadvantages. As such, in Chapter 1, different novel anthropometric parameters and cardiovascular risk factors among obesity adults are compared and evaluated.

Chapter 2 describes a study of children aged 0-12 years conducted in the Middle Senegal River Valley (MISOES) in 1957-1958. This study was based on representative samples of children in urban and rural areas and included measurements of weight, height, arm circumference, and more. These measurements were compared with American standards and showed an overwhelming anthropometric deficit compared with standards. This study is examined in the context of other studies conducted in the region as well as in connection with economic development in the valley. Chapter 3 describes the various methods of assessing body fat and their application for obese individuals to predict the risk of Coronary Heart Disease (CHD), and Chapter 4 reviews the effect of different modalities of physical exercise on anthropometric measurements and body composition in different populations of older adults.

Chapter 1 - Overweight and obesity are common problems in developed countries and becoming increasingly problematic in developing countries. The worldwide prevalence of obesity has more than doubled, an estimated 39% of the world's adult population aged over 18 years were overweight and 13% were obese over the past 3 decades. Obesity is defined as an abnormal or excessive accumulation of body fat that may impair health. Obesity is the causal component in the pathogenesis of type 2 diabetes mellitus (T2DM), cardiovascular diseases (CVD), and several cancers. However, obesity is preventable and early detection may play an important role in overcoming the condition and associated metabolic complications. The development of these comorbidities is proportionate to BMI and obesity is considered as an independent risk factor for cardiovascular events. Although obesity is generally accepted as a risk factor for cardiovascular events, some studies showed that obesity could decrease mortality. This association seems blunted in some chronic condition with obese individuals presenting with a survival advantage over their counterparts, a phenomenon termed the "obesity paradox." The use of body mass index (BMI) as a health risk phenotype has several limitations because BMI does not accurately depict different components of body composition and is therefore unable to predict the prognostic effect of individual tissues. Other widely used anthropometric indices of central obesity are waist circumference (WC), waist to hip ratio (WHR), waist to height ratio (WHtR), and others. Each index has both advantages and disadvantages. Hitherto, no anthropometric measurement for obesity satisfies the criteria of being accurate, precise, accessible, and widely acceptable. The purpose of this review was to compare and evaluate the associations and the optimal cut-off values between different novel anthropometric parameters and cardiovascular risk factors among obesity adults.

Chapter 2 - The anthropometry of children aged 0-12 years was studied during the multiple objectives survey conducted in the Middle Senegal River Valley (MISOES) in 1957-1958. This survey was based on two representative samples, in urban areas (769 children) and in rural areas (1240 children). Several measurements were taken: weight, height, arm circumference, triceps skinfold, subscapular skinfold, sub-iliac crest height, biacromial breadth, biiliac breadth. They were compared with American standards. Data show an overwhelming anthropometric deficit compared with standards, and complex interactions with age, gender, and place of residence. The average deficit, expressed as the percentage of reference values were: 80.6% for weight, 95.5% for height, 91.7% for body mass index (BMI), 78.6% for body surface area; it was more marked for triceps skinfold (67.6%) and for subscapular skinfold (66.3%), but less for arm circumference (84.9%) and for muscle circumference (87.7%); it was also marked for biacromial breadth (90.5%) and for biiliac breadth (91.9%), although keeping approximately constant the acromial-iliac ratio. Overall, deficits were more marked among children 1-2 years old, as well as among the 9-12 years old. Gender differences were not pronounced, but boys were somewhat disadvantaged before age 3 years, while girls were in greater deficit at age 9-12 years. Differences by place of residence were small and complex: deficits were higher in rural areas for skinfolds, but higher in urban areas for arm- and muscle- circumference. Results from the MISOES survey were put into perspective by comparing them with other studies also conducted in Senegal among under-five children: Niakhar (1983-1984) and DHS surveys (1993-2017). The relationships with economic development in the valley are discussed.

Chapter 3 - Overweight and obesity are associated with an increased risk of cardiovascular disease and considered to be one of the leading risk factors for mortality. Numerous health risks are associated with different types of fat distribution patterns. It has been found that central obesity is associated with a number of metabolic abnormalities such as hypertension, hyperinsulinemia, and hyperlipidemia. Anthropometry is a science which deals with the measurements of human size, shape and proportion. It encompasses a variety of human body measurements such as weight, stature, skinfold thickness, circumferences, limb lengths, and breadths. Various anthropometric methods are available for the assessment of body fat. The general and central obesity anthropometric measures used for assessing adiposity-related risk include body mass index, waist circumference, hip circumference, waist-to-hip ratio, waist-to-stature ratio and body adiposity index. Central obesity measures including waist circumference and waist-hip ratio are considered better markers of the risk of Coronary Heart Disease (CHD) than body mass index among obese people. Fat distribution determines the cardio-metabolic problems associated with adiposity rather than total body fat. This can be due to an imbalance in the production of inflammatory and anti-inflammatory adipokines. Anthropometric measurements are among the simplest, non-invasive and low-cost methods to measure obesity and the risk of CHD among mass populations. The present chapter deals with the various methods used for assessing body fat and their application for obese individuals to predict the risk of CHD.

Chapter 4 - Age-related changes regarding anthropometry or body composition such as the decrease in muscle mass, the increase in body fat, and the loss of bone mass have important systemic implications and are significant contributors to functional limitation in the old age. However, there is evidence supporting the positive role of physical exercise and active lifestyles in these variables. The purpose of this chapter is to review the effect of different modalities of physical exercise on anthropometric measurements and body composition in different populations of older adults. Public health policies aimed to prescribe exercise programs must account for these specific implications.

In: Anthropometry
Editor: Sébastien Legrand

ISBN: 978-1-53619-269-8
© 2021 Nova Science Publishers, Inc.

Chapter 1

ASSOCIATION BETWEEN NOVEL ANTHROPOMETRIC PARAMETERS AND CARDIOVASCULAR RISK FACTORS AMONG OBESE ADULTS

Wattana Leowattana[*]
Department of Clinical Tropical Medicine,
Faculty of Tropical Medicine, Mahidol University,
Bangkok, Thailand

ABSTRACT

Overweight and obesity are common problems in developed countries and becoming increasingly problematic in developing countries. The worldwide prevalence of obesity has more than doubled, an estimated 39% of the world's adult population aged over 18 years were overweight and 13% were obese over the past 3 decades. Obesity is defined as an abnormal or excessive accumulation of body fat that may impair health. Obesity is the causal component in the pathogenesis of

---

[*] Corresponding Author's E-mail: wattana.leo@mahidol.ac.th.

type 2 diabetes mellitus (T2DM), cardiovascular diseases (CVD), and several cancers. However, obesity is preventable and early detection may play an important role in overcoming the condition and associated metabolic complications. The development of these comorbidities is proportionate to BMI and obesity is considered as an independent risk factor for cardiovascular events. Although obesity is generally accepted as a risk factor for cardiovascular events, some studies showed that obesity could decrease mortality. This association seems blunted in some chronic condition with obese individuals presenting with a survival advantage over their counterparts, a phenomenon termed the "obesity paradox." The use of body mass index (BMI) as a health risk phenotype has several limitations because BMI does not accurately depict different components of body composition and is therefore unable to predict the prognostic effect of individual tissues. Other widely used anthropometric indices of central obesity are waist circumference (WC), waist to hip ratio (WHR), waist to height ratio (WHtR), and others. Each index has both advantages and disadvantages. Hitherto, no anthropometric measurement for obesity satisfies the criteria of being accurate, precise, accessible, and widely acceptable. The purpose of this review was to compare and evaluate the associations and the optimal cut-off values between different novel anthropometric parameters and cardiovascular risk factors among obesity adults.

Keywords: overweight, obesity, cardiovascular risk factors, cardiovascular diseases, type 2 diabetes mellitus, anthropometric parameter, BMI, WC, WHR, and WHtR

INTRODUCTION

Obesity is an abnormal or excessive accumulation of body fat that impair health [1]. Humans acquire all energy from ingested food and drink, store it as high-energy molecules, and expend it during basal metabolic functions, activity, and thermogenesis. Body fat mass increases when energy intake exceeds energy expenditure. A positive energy balance will result in obesity for an extended period [2]. Nowadays, obesity has been a health problem of growing significance around the globe. Its prevalence is increasing in both developed and developing countries. Obesity is an essential factor in developing metabolic syndrome and cardiovascular disease and is also a substantial contributing cause of muscle loss [3]. In general, we usually diagnosed obesity by assessing body mass index (BMI), a proxy measure of body fat that relied on the person's weight adjusted for height. Obesity is categorized in different classes, accordingly with BMI increase. While a BMI between 18.50 – 24.99 kg/m² defines, as usual, BMI between 25 - 29.99 kg/m² defines as overweight, those with BMI > 30 kg/m² are categorized as obese. In the obesity group, a BMI between 30 - 34.99 kg/m² defines as class I obesity (obese), between 35 - 39.99 kg/m² defines as class II obesity (severely obese), and > 40 kg/m² defines as class III obesity (morbidly obese) [4] (Figure 1).

As of 2016, the World Health Organization (WHO) reported that approximately 39% of the global population had a BMI > 25 kg/m² and was considered overweight and obese [5]. Numerous studies have demonstrated a relationship between obesity and cardiovascular diseases [6]. The association between obesity and hypertension, diabetes mellitus, dyslipidemias, and sleep apnea syndrome has also been shown to increase the incidence of cardiovascular disorders (CVDs) [7]. CVDs are serious circulatory diseases that endanger human health and are the main cause of mortality worldwide. Nearly 17.9 million people around the world died from CVDs, accounting for 31% of global deaths. It is demonstrated that adults characterized by excessive fatty tissue and ectopic fat stores have a higher risk of CVDs [8]. Long-standing evidence has demonstrated the linkage between obesity and increased risk of hypertension, type-2 diabetes mellitus (T2DM), and dyslipidemia, major risk factors for CVDs [9, 10, 11]. However, the definition of obesity remains controversial, and discrepancies in anthropometric parameters and may lead to inaccurate assessment for CVD risk factors. BMI is a generally recognized anthropometric index of obesity, regardless of age, sex, or ethnicity, and several epidemiological studies have confirmed that BMI can predict CVD risk factors [12]. Although obesity is generally accepted as a risk factor for CVDs, some studies showed that obesity could decrease mortality. This association seems blunted in some chronic conditions with obese individuals presenting with a survival advantage over their counterparts, and a phenomenon termed the "obesity paradox." In 2002, Gruberg and colleagues conducted a study of 9,633 consecutive obese patients with coronary artery disease (CAD) who underwent percutaneous coronary intervention (PCI). The patients were divided into three groups regarding to BMI: normal, BMI between 18.5 and 24.9 kg/m^2 (n = 1,923); overweight, BMI between 25 and 30 kg/m^2 (n = 4,813); and obese, BMI >30 kg/m^2 (n = 2,897). They reported that in patients with known CAD who underwent PCI, very lean patients (BMI <18.5 kg/m^2) and those with normal BMI were at the highest risk for in-hospital complications, cardiac death, and increased one-year mortality [13]. It was defined that when obesity and CVDs coexist, individuals with class I obesity presented a more favorable prognosis compared to individuals who are normal or underweight [14, 15]. Several studies have shown a protective role of obesity for overall and cardiovascular (CV) mortality in patients affected by coronary heart disease (CHD), heart failure (HF), atrial fibrillation (AF), end-stage renal disease (ESRD), chronic obstructive pulmonary disease (COPD) and T2DM. In 2013, Flegal and colleagues conducted a meta-analysis that studied the hazard ratios (HRs) of all-cause mortality for overweight and obesity relative to normal weight in the general population. They evaluated 97 prospective studies, including a total of 2.88 million participants and more than 270,000 deaths. They concluded that relative to normal weight, both obesity grades 2 and 3 were associated with significantly higher all-cause mortality. Grade 1 obesity was not associated with higher mortality, and overweight was associated with significantly lower all-cause mortality [16]. Recently, Zhang and colleagues conducted a meta-analysis study by recruited ten studies that included 96,424 patients [59,263 had HF with preserved ejection fraction (HFpEF), and 37,161 had HF with reduced EF (HFrEF)] to evaluate an inverse relationship between BMI and the mortality. They found that for patients with HF, the relation between BMI and mortality is U-shaped with a similar nadir of risk for HFpEF and HFrEF at a BMI of 32-33 kg/m^2 [17].

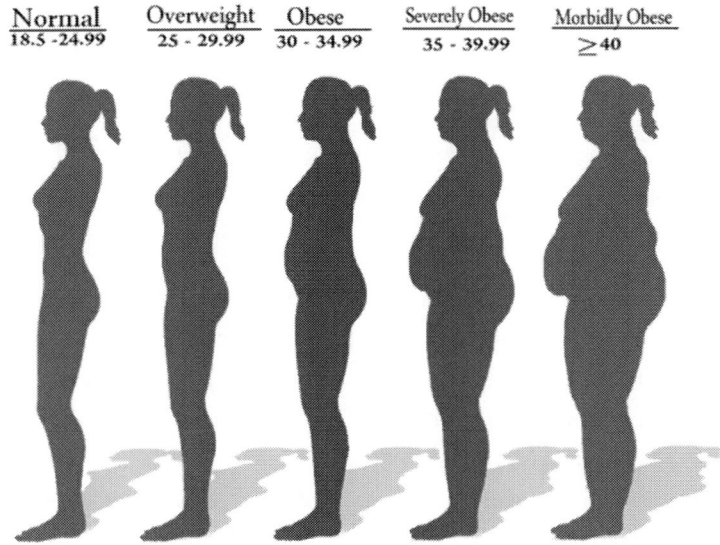

Figure 1. The classification of overweight and obesity is defined by body mass index (BMI), regardless of age, sex, or ethnicity.

NOVEL ANTHROPOMETRIC PARAMETERS

Traditionally, overweight and obesity have been assessed based on excess body weight, most commonly relative to height, assuming that excess body fat is recognized to be present at higher levels of body weight. However, many heavier individuals may be classified as overweight or obese based on high muscle mass levels. Bodyweight is not a measure of body composition and does not differentiate between body composition's significant components (fat mass vs. fat-free mass). The amount of body fat in different body regions also varies considerably between individuals and is a significant factor in determining health risk [18, 19]. Notably, BMI does not distinguish between body fat and lean mass and therefore overestimates fatness among those who are muscular [20, 21, 22]. Dwivedi and colleagues recently conducted a systematic review and meta-analysis regarding the association between obesity and cardiovascular outcomes. They found a U-shaped pattern between BMI levels and risk of HF mortality, SCD, and CVD mortality in specific CVD populations, with the highest risk in underweight subjects followed by normal BMI subjects and lowest in overweight, with a slightly higher risk in obese followed by morbidly obese individuals [23]. These findings confirmed the obesity paradox related to the most popular anthropometric index, BMI. However, measures of central obesity, principally waist-hip-height ratio (WHHtR), waist-height ratio (WHtR), ponderal index (PI), waist-thigh ratio (WTR), sagittal abdominal diameter-height ratio (SADHtR), body adiposity index (BAI), and C-index, which more accurately describe the distribution of body fat compared with BMI, have been suggested to be more closely associated with subsequent morbidity and mortality [24, 25, 26, 27, 28, 29, 30] (Table 1). An ideal anthropometric measure for defining adiposity and obesity should be both simple and accurate. Several novel anthropometric parameters used complex calculations to evaluate the fatness in obese adults. Moreover, some anthropometric parameters relied upon several body measurements that were both complex and difficult to measure with precision. The lack of simplicity to calculate is likely to be a significant drawback in applying some of the novel anthropometric parameters in the real world as a screening tool for overweight and obesity in primary and secondary healthcare settings.

CELLULAR PATHOPHYSIOLOGY IN OBESITY

There are several mechanisms responsible for the harmful effects of obesity on the CV system. It is accepted that obesity arises from an energy imbalance when calories utilized is less than what is intake [31]. The human body responded and adapted to excess energy intake once it exceeds that of the body's metabolic needs at the cellular level. Once BW increases more than 170% of the average level, adipocyte size could increase as doubles of standard, and its function may be altered [32, 33]. The driving factors of adipocyte hyperplasia are the recruitment of adipogenic progenitors and growth factors [insulin-like growth factor-1 (IGF-1), IGF-binding proteins, tumor necrosis factor (TNF)-α, angiotensin

II, and macrophage colony-stimulating factor. When the BW increases to the advanced level, the hypertrophied adipocytes undergo apoptosis, cell necrosis, and fibrosis, which further induces an inflammatory pathway and adipose tissue dysfunction [34]. The macrophage recruitment to adipose tissue will intensify insulin resistance (IR) after initiating the inflammatory response. The pro-inflammatory cytokines reduced ABCA1 and ABCG1 expression in macrophages and decreased phospholipids' uptake and cholesterol from the cells to high-density lipoproteins (HDL). Moreover, lipid metabolism is also affected by adipokines, leptin, adiponectin, and increasing serum free fatty acid levels [35, 36]. The vascular endothelial cells of adipose tissue in obesity were also activated. These cells aid in the inflammatory process through the expression of adhesion molecules and chemotactic factors. These further induce inflammatory cells and end up with adipocyte dysfunction. The increased pro-inflammatory cytokines state, and endocrine abnormalities caused by obesity likely contribute to escalated risks for CVDs [37].

CV Risk Factors in Obesity

Hypertension

Hypertension (HTN) occurs in around 50% of overweight and obese patients and is directly associated with the development of CVDs. The Physicians' Health Study demonstrated a strong association between higher BMI and the risk of HTN in a large cohort of male physicians followed for a median of 14.5 years (1 unit of BMI will increase about 8% of CVD risk) [38]. The increased IR, sodium retention, vascular endothelial hyperactive, sympathetic nervous system activation, and hyperinsulinemia could induce the development of HTN in obese patients [39]. Multiple structural changes are another contributing factor in hypertensive obesity. Obese patients with HTN usually increased left ventricular mass (LVM), higher stroke volume, and higher cardiac output than people with normal blood pressure [40]. The adaptation of the cardiac structure of obese patients with HTN depended on where excess fat is carried. In obese patients with central fat distribution, concentric LV remodeling and left ventricular hypertrophy (LVH) were developed. The ventricular walls were thickened with increased LVM. In comparison, those with peripheral fat distribution developed eccentric LVH. The ventricular walls were dilatated with increased LVM [41, 42]. A sustained modest weight loss substantially lowers the long-term risk of hypertension in overweight and obese adults [43].

Table 1. Novel anthropometric parameters

Indices	Measurement	Cut-off	References
Waist-hip-height ratio (WHHtR)	WC (m) x Ht (m) HC (m)	NR	Song et al., Finland [24]
Waist-height ratio (WHtR)	WC (cm) Ht (cm)	0.50	Hsieh et al., Japan [25]
Ponderal index (PI)	Wt (kg) Ht (cm)^3	Hypertension, Pre-hypertension M = 14.45, 13.69 F = 16.38, 17.65	Ononamadu et al., Nigeria [26]
Waist-thigh ratio (WTR)	WC (cm) TC (cm)	NR	Li et al., USA [27]
Sagittal abdominal diameter-height ratio (SADHtR)	SAD (cm) Ht (cm)	NR	Carlsson et al., Sweden [28]
Body adiposity index (BAI)	HC (cm) - 18 Ht (cm)$^{1.5}$	Cardiometabolic abnormalities >1 M = 26.39 F = 31.29 Cardiometabolic abnormalities >2 M = 27.82 F = 31.29	Fu et al., China [29]
Conicity index (C-index)	WC (m) $\sqrt[0.109]{BW}$ (kg) Ht (m)	NR	Kommuri et al., USA [30]

BW = body weight, F = female, HC = hip circumference, Ht = height, M = male, NR = not reported, SAD = sagittal abdominal diameter, TC = thigh circumference, WC = waist circumference, Wt = weight.

Metabolic Syndrome

Metabolic syndrome (MetS) is the cluster of clinical and metabolic factors that increase the risk for T2DM, CAD, and stroke. The associated risk factors include central obesity, dyslipidemias, hypertension, hypercoagulable state, and IR [44]. The persons with MetS, the risk of developing T2DM is five times greater, and the risk of stroke and myocardial infarction is three times higher as compared to healthy subjects [45]. Moreover, MetS have also been associated with hepatic steatosis and non-alcoholic fatty liver disease (NAFLD), hypogonadism, polycystic ovary syndrome (PCOS), obstructive sleep apnea, vascular dementia, Alzheimer's disease, pancreatic cancers, and colorectal cancers [46, 47]. The phenotypic components of MetS, combined with the cellular changes, lead to the development of a pro-inflammatory state and the progression of atherosclerosis [48]. Obese men with MetS have an increased risk of all-cause mortality (OR = 1.55, 95% CI = 1.14 - 2.11) and CVD mortality (OR = 2.83, 95% CI = 1.70 - 4.72) when compared to their normal-weight counterparts (OR = 1.11, 95% CI = 0.75 - 1.17, and OR = 1.80, 95% CI = 1.10 - 2.97, respectively) [49]. Isomaa and colleagues conducted the study to evaluate the prevalence of the CV risk associated with the MetS in 4,483 subjects aged 35-70 years in Finland and Sweden. They found a 3-fold increased risk of CVD and stroke in both men and women with MetS. Moreover, several studies reported that metabolically healthy obesity had a significantly lower risk for all-cause, cancer, and CVD mortality than metabolically abnormal obese individuals [50, 51, 52, 53]. Studies and pharmacological trials strongly support the critical role of lifestyle interventions involving weight reduction and the adoption of a healthy diet, accompanied by anti-obesity drugs, to decrease or delay the progression of MetS and its complications. Physical activity is the most critical lifestyle intervention that can substantially improve insulin sensitivity, glycemic control, and cardiovascular remodeling [54].

Dyslipidemia

Dyslipidemia is a well-known risk factor for a significant contributor to CVD and myocardial infarction (MI). The increased levels of low-density–lipoprotein cholesterol (LDL-C), total cholesterol (TC), and decreased levels of high-density–lipoprotein cholesterol (HDL-C) are well-established contributors to CVD [55, 56]. Hypertriglyceridemia is also an independent risk factor for CVD [57, 58]. The typical dyslipidemia of obesity consists of increased triglycerides (TG) and free fatty acid (FFA), decreased HDL-C with HDL dysfunction, and standard or slightly increased LDL-C with increased small dense LDL. The hypertriglyceridemia may be the primary cause of the other lipid abnormalities since it will lead to delayed clearance of the TG-rich lipoproteins and formation of small dense LDL [59]. It has been demonstrated that LDL particle size rather than total level has a stronger association with atherogenicity. Hence, larger particles may be less atherogenic [60]. Whereas all obesity-associated dyslipidemia components have been linked with increased CV risk, low HDL-C was one of the most potent risk factors. The strong inverse relationship between HDL-C levels and CV disease incidence has been demonstrated in several extensive observational studies. Even if LDL-C levels are below 70 mg/dl, low HDL-C is still associated with an increased CV disease risk [61]. Plasma FFA is derived from lipolysis of TG-rich lipoproteins within the circulation and intracellular lipolysis in adipose tissue. The increase in plasma FFA and obesity-induced inflammation plays a crucial role in developing IR [62]. Various FFAs are cytotoxic, and their cytotoxicity depends on the type. Saturated fatty acids (SFA), arachidonic acid, and linoleic acid can mediate a diet-induced inflammation by stimulation, producing pro-inflammatory cytokines like IL-1, IL-6, and TNF-α [63].

Heart Failure

Obesity induces hemodynamic and humoral changes associated with functional and structural cardiac remodeling, which ultimately results in HF development. In obese subjects, excessive adipose tissue accumulation is related to increased blood volume and reduced systemic vascular resistance, which results in augmentation of cardiac output [64]. Fat-free mass in obese individuals is one of the most critical factors in developing a hypercirculatory state in obese patients. Because the heart rate is slightly increased in obese subjects, the primary reason for increased cardiac output in obesity lies in LV stroke volume. The cardiac effort, particularly LV effort in obese patients, overcame values predicted for those with average body weight due to increased LV stroke work. LV end-diastolic pressure and pulmonary capillary wedge pressure are generally elevated in moderate-to-severely obese patients. In 2002, Kenchaiah and colleagues reported 5,881 patients in the Framingham Heart Study that BMI correlates with HF risk in a dose-dependent condition. When one unit of BMI increased, the HF risk for men will escalate by 5% and for women by 7% after adjusting for demographics and other known risk factors [65]. The larger Physicians' Health Study of 21,094 men without known CAD was conducted in 2009 by Kenchaiah and colleagues and found a positive correlation between BMI and HF risk for overweight and obese physicians. The overweight participants had a 49% increase in HF risk than lean participants, and obese participants had a 180% increase in HF risk [66]. In 2010, Hu and colleagues conducted a study cohort that included 59,178 Finnish participants free of HF at baseline. They evaluated the associations of physical activity and different anthropometries of adiposity with HF risk. They found an independent association between overweight and abdominal obesity with an increased risk of HF. Moreover, moderate or high intensities of physical activity were associated with a reduced risk of HF. The protective effect of physical activity on HF risk is observed at all BMI levels [67]. In Sweden, Levitan and colleagues conducted a prospective cohort of 80,630 Swedish men and women who were high BMI, WC, WHtI to evaluate the association between obesity and risk of hospitalization and mortality in HF patients. They found that the strength of the association between BMI and HF events declined with age. They concluded that higher BMI, higher WC, and higher WHtI associated with a higher risk of HF hospitalization and mortality [68]. A recent study included 22,681 participants from four community-based cohorts and examined the incidence of HFpEF and HFrEF during the median follow-up period of 12 years. They reported that greater BMI was associated with a higher risk of HFpEF in comparison with HFrEF, and this relationship was more pronounced among women when compared with men. Additionally, IR was only associated with HFpEF, but not HFrEF [69].

Atrial Fibrillation

Obesity is significantly associated with developing AF and is estimated to be responsible for a 50% increased AF incidence [70]. Wang and colleagues reported a 4% increase in risk for AF per 1 unit increase in BMI. They calculated the risk after a mean follow-up of 13.7 years. In 2014, Frost and colleagues conducted a prospective cohort study to evaluate the relationship between the risk of AF with body fat, body fat location, and lean body mass in 55,273 men and women, 50-64 years of age. The results showed higher body fat and higher lean body mass associated with a higher risk of AF at any measured location during 13.5 years follow-up [71]. Schmidt and colleagues reported that overweight and obese young men have a 2-fold risk of AF compared to lean comparatives [72]. In 2014, Özcan and colleagues reported that resistin, mainly secreted from lipid cells, is linked to T2DM and obesity, correlated with paroxysmal and persistent AF [73]. Numerous studies reported that obesity independently predicts paroxysmal progression to permanent AF [74, 75, 76]. AF in patients with obesity comprised complex pathophysiological mechanisms that remain poorly understood. The crucial factors were hypertension, T2DM, MetS, CAD, obstructive sleep apnea (OSA), and left atrial remodeling [77].

WAIST-HIP-HEIGHT RATIO (WHHtR)

Song et al. firstly described WC to HC to height ratio (WHHtR) and is calculated as the ratio between WC, HC, and height (Table 1) [24]. In 2013, Song and colleagues conducted a prospective cohort study to investigate the relationship between CVD mortality and different obesity indicators, including BMI, WC, WHR, waist-to-stature ratio (WSR), a body shape index (ABSI), and WHHtR in 46,651 Europeans aged 24 - 99 years. They found that 3,435 participants died, specifically 1,409 participants died from CVD. The results demonstrated that all obesity indicators were positively associated with increased risk of CVD mortality, with HRs (95% confidence intervals) per standard deviation increase of 1.19 (1.12-1.27) for BMI, 1.29 (1.21-1.37) for WC, 1.28 (1.20-1.36) for WHR, 1.35 (1.27-1.44) for WSR, 1.34 (1.26-1.44) for ABSI and 1.34 (1.25-1.42) for WHHtR in men and 1.37 (1.24-1.51), 1.49 (1.34-1.65), 1.45 (1.31-1.60), 1.52 (1.37-1.69), 1.32 (1.18-1.48) and 1.45 (1.31-1.61) in women, respectively. The prediction was stronger with abdominal obesity indicators than with BMI or ABSI. They concluded that abdominal obesity indicators such as WC, WHR, WSR, and WHHtR, are stronger predictors for CVD mortality than general obesity indicators of BMI [24]. In 2014, Fu and colleagues conducted a descriptive cross-sectional study to evaluate the relationship between anthropometric indices and cardiometabolic abnormalities in a Chinese community-dwelling population. They recruited 4,868 residents through a large health check-up program in Beijing. The authors recommended a cut-off WHHtR value of 0.51 in males and 0.53 in females for the presence of one or more cardiometabolic abnormalities. The results showed a significant association between WHHtR with cardiometabolic abnormalities, T2DM, and dyslipidemia. However, they found that WHR, when compared with other anthropometric indexes, can reflect the compound risk of different cardiometabolic abnormalities and the greatest potential to be widely applied in clinical practice [78]. Song and colleagues compared WHHtR and other anthropometric indices' ability to predict CVD mortality in a longitudinal cohort study involving 50,093 adults from 12 prospective studies conducted in 4 different European countries (Finland, Sweden, Turkey, and the UK). The results revealed that WC (HR: 1.29–1.49), WHR (HR: 1.28–1.45), WHtR (HR: 1.35–1.52), and WHHtR (HR: 1.37–1.45) were stronger predictors for CVD mortality than a body shape index (ABSI) (HR: 1.32–1.34) or BMI (HR: 1.19–1.37) [24]. The studies by Carlsson and colleagues reported similar results. They conducted a study cohort of 3,741 adults without CVD followed up for 11 years. They found that WHHtR (HR: 1.20) and WHR (HR: 1.14) were the best predictors of CVD in normal-weight women and among overweight and obese individuals. The WHHtR was the strongest predictor after adjustments for CVD risk factors in men [79]. In 2017, Hardy and colleagues used Atherosclerosis Risk in Communities (ARIC) study data from 12,121 participants aged 45-64 years without diabetes at baseline who were followed for over 11 years. The anthropometric measures included ABSI, BAI, BMI, WC, WHR, WHtR, and WHHtR. Among White and Black males and females, BMI, WC, WHR, and WHtR were comparable in discriminating cases from non-cases of T2DM. ABSI, BAI, and WHHtR were inferior discriminators of incident T2DM across all race-gender groups. They concluded that BMI and three anthropometric measures (WC, WHR, WHtR) were the best anthropometric discriminators of incident T2DM across all race-gender groups in the ARIC cohort [80].

WAIST-HEIGHT RATIO (WHtR)

In 1995, Hsieh and Yoshinaga introduced the waist-height ratio (WHtR) as a useful predictor for Japanese men's CHD risk factors. They studied 3,131 men who underwent a routine health examination. They found that BMI, WHR, and WHtR were significantly associated with all of the risk factors. According to the multiple regression analysis results for WHtR and BMI, BMI was not significantly associated with fasting blood glucose, HbA1c, cholesterol levels, or the risk factor morbidity index, whereas WHtR was significantly associated with the variables. They concluded that WHtR, an index of abdominal obesity, maybe a better predictor of multiple CHD risk factors in men [25]. In 2010, Browning and colleagues conducted a systematic review of WHtR as a screening tool for predicting cardiovascular disease and diabetes. They included seventy-eight studies exploring WHtR and WC or BMI as predictors of diabetes and CVD, published between 1950 and 2008. Twenty-two prospective analyses showed that WHtR and WC were better significant predictors of cardiometabolic outcomes than BMI. Observations from cross-sectional analysis, forty-four studies in adults, and thirteen studies in children supported these predictions. Receiver operator characteristic (ROC) analysis revealed a mean area under ROC (AUROC) values of 0.704, 0.693, and 0.671 for WHtR, WC, and BMI, respectively. Mean boundary values for WHtR, covering all cardiometabolic outcomes, from studies in fourteen different countries and Caucasian, Asian, and Central American subjects, were 0.50 for men and women. WHtR and WC were similar predictors of diabetes and CVD, both being stronger than BMI [81]. In 2012, Ashwell and colleagues conducted a systematic review and meta-analysis to evaluate the screening potential of WHtR and WC for adult cardiometabolic risk in people of different nationalities and to compare both with BMI. They included Thirty-one papers in their study involving more than 300,000 adults in several ethnic groups. They found that WHtR had significantly greater discriminatory power compared with BMI. Compared with BMI, WC improved discrimination of adverse outcomes by 3% (P < 0.05) and WHtR improved discrimination by 4-5% over BMI (P < 0.01). Statistical analysis of the within-study difference in AUC demonstrated WHtR to be significantly better than WC for diabetes, hypertension, CVD, and all outcomes (p < 0.005) in men and women. They concluded that the results showed the superiority of WHtR over WC and BMI for detecting cardiometabolic risk factors in both sexes. WHtR should, therefore, be considered as a screening tool [82]. In 2016, Corrêa and colleagues conducted a systematic literature review to elucidate the performance of the WHtR in identifying obesity and predicting non-communicable diseases in the elderly population. They included sixteen papers in their study involving 357,171 adults. The results showed that WHtR is a valid anthropometric index to diagnose obesity among the elderly and is considered a good indicator in predicting risk factors for

CVDs, MetS, and diabetes compared to BMI, WC, and WHR. The association between WHtR and chronic diseases differed among age groups and was considered the best predictor among younger elderly persons compared to the older ones. They concluded that WHtR alone or combined with WC was the best anthropometric index in predicting cardiovascular risk factors than the other indices [83]. Recently, Rangel-Baltazar and colleagues conducted a study to describe the association between a high WHtR and cardiovascular risk (CVR) indicators among Mexican adults and examine sex and age interaction on the association. They found that over 90% of participants had high WHtR and were at greater risk for dyslipidemias, HTN, and IR compared to those that had low WHtR. Prevalence ratio (PR) for men with high WHtR were between 1.3 to 2.3 for dyslipidemias, 3.4 for HTN, and 7.6 for IR; among women were between 1.8 to 2.4 for dyslipidemias and HTN and 5.9 for IR ($p < 0.05$). They concluded that high WHtR is associated with CVR factors in Mexican adults [84]. In 2020, Lo and colleagues conducted a study to compare the association between obesity indices and chronic diseases at baseline and the subsequent mortality risk among 21,109 US adults. They found that Elevated WHtR, elevated WC, and BMI were associated with higher odds of hypertension (OR: 1.37-2.13), dyslipidemia (OR: 1.06-1.75), and diabetes (OR: 1.40-3.16). Moreover, WHtR had significantly better discriminatory power to predict cardiometabolic health than BMI, especially for diabetes. They concluded that WHtR and WC appeared to be the better indicators for cardiometabolic health than BMI. However, BMI had a stronger and inverse association with a greater risk of all-cause mortality among older females [85].

PONDERAL INDEX (PI)

Fay and colleagues originally described the PI as a measure of intrauterine growth retardation in infants. It is derived by dividing weight in kilograms by (height) 3 in centimeters [86]. In 2017, Ononamadu and colleagues conducted a study to compare eight anthropometric indices of obesity: BMI, PI, WC, HC, WHR, WHtR, and BAI as correlates and potential predictors risk of HTN and pre-hypertension in 912 Nigerian participants. They found that BMI, WHtR, WC, and PI were the best predictors of hypertension risk and BMI, WC, and PI of pre-hypertension risk. Moreover, the combination of high-performing anthropometric indices did not improve their performance. The PI had low discriminatory power for both conditions [86]. In 2019, Zaniqueli and colleagues conducted a cross-sectional study with 1,149 participants (53.2% male), aged 6 to 18 years, to compare the PI with BMI-for-age z-scores transformed (BMIz) in estimating body fat levels and classifying obesity in children and adolescents in a Brazilian urban population. They found that PI and BMIz were similar stability indexes from childhood to adolescence for both boys and girls. They concluded that PI is a promising index for replacing BMIz in children and adolescents due to reduced false diagnosis of obesity. The PI may be applied for adult obesity evaluation [87].

WAIST-THIGH RATIO (WTR)

WC to TC ratio (WTR) is defined as the ratio between WC and mid-TC. In 2010, Li and colleagues conducted a study to examine whether WTR performed better than WHtR, WHR, WC, or BMI concerning diabetes among 6,277 US adults. They found that WTR performed better than the other four indices in men, and WTR performed similarly to WHtR, WHR, and WC, but better than BMI in women for the association with diabetes [27]. Lu and colleagues reported the study results to evaluate the association of peripheral vascular disease (PVD) with WTR and WC in 2010. The study population consisted of 5,057 adults aged 40 years or older. They found that WTR was strongly associated with PVD in men, among women; a strong linear trend was found indicating a significant association between WTR and PVD. They concluded that WTR is associated with PVD in men and women. In contrast, WC is associated with PVD in women but not in men [88]. In 2018, Beraldo and colleagues conducted a study to evaluate adiposity indexes and cut-off value associated with predictors of CVD risk in HIV patients on highly active antiretroviral therapy (HAART). They found that WC and WHtR showed the best performances for central adiposity evaluation. They concluded that the indexes of central adiposity presented excellent associations with predictors of CVD risk, and the use of the specific cut-offs could contribute to the early identification of increased risk of CVDs and will enabling early interventions [89].

SAGITTAL ABDOMINAL DIAMETER-HEIGHT RATIO (SADHtR)

The sagittal abdominal diameter to height ratio (SADHtR) was firstly reported in 1997 by Kumlin et al. [90]. They showed that shows that the SAD and the SADHtR had similar correlations with the Framingham index. They concluded that conclude that the SADHtR may be a useful indicator of coronary risk. Furthermore, SADHtR was used to predict ischemic CVD risk in an 11-year longitudinal cohort study comprising 3,471 Swedish people. In 2013, Carlsson and colleagues conducted a study to compare novel and established anthropometric indexes in predicting CVD and determine whether they improve risk prediction beyond classical risk factors in a cohort study of 60-year-old men and women. The SAD was measured as the perpendicular distance between the table and top of the body at the iliac crest level in a supine position, measured after a normal expiration, using a ruler and spirit level. The SADHtR was a strong predictor of ischemic CVD risk in the cohort. BMI (HR: 0.99–1.08), WC (HR: 0.99–1.07), and WHtR (HR: 1.04–1.12) were weaker predictors than SAD (HR: 1.05–1.16) and SADHtR (HR: 1.10–1.19) in predicting ischemic CVD [28]. In 2000, Bertin and colleagues conducted a study to get accurate measurements of visceral adipose tissue (VAT) using dual-energy X-ray absorptiometry (DXA). They compared DXA and anthropometric data and their combinations to the VAT area calculated from a computed tomography (CT) single scan in 71 overweight subjects.

They concluded that SADHtR was closely related to VAT (r = 0.94 for women and 0.88 for men) and showed better performance in predicting the VAT area without measuring it by CT [91]. In 2018, Kahn and Cheng conducted a study to evaluate the association of SADHtR, WHtR, and BMI with fasting insulin, triglycerides, and three biomarkers of IR levels in 4,398 adults. They found that the RRs for WHtR were consistent between those for SADHtR and BMI. The top 25% of IR among US adults was above adiposity thresholds of 0.140 for SADHtR, 0.606 for WHtR, or 29.6 kg/m² for BMI. They concluded that the relative abdominal size rather than relative weight might better define adiposity associated with homeostatic IR [92].

BODY ADIPOSITY INDEX (BAI)

Body adiposity index (BAI) is an anthropometric parameter derived from HC (cm)/height (m)$^{1.5}$ − 18. It was first described by Bergman et al. as a direct estimate of percentage adiposity [93]. Fu and colleagues found a significant correlation between BAI and cardiometabolic abnormalities (hypertension, T2DM, and dyslipidemia) in a descriptive cross-sectional study, including 4,868 subjects. They found that BAI is not a more useful identifier of cardiometabolic abnormalities than other indices [29]. Moreover, Lam and colleagues also reported that the associations of BAI and cardiometabolic abnormalities were weaker than traditional anthropometric parameters [94]. In 2015, Belarmino and colleagues conducted a study to evaluate BAI's performance in estimating body fat percentage (BF%) in severely obese patients. They found that BAI did not provide an accurate estimate of BF% and has been reported to poorly predict body fat indices in obese women and athletes [95]. In 2016, D'Elia and colleagues conducted a study to compare BMI and BAI's predictive role on the risk of HTN, BP changes, and subclinical organ damage in 350 adult men participating in the Olivetti Heart Study. They found that BAI and BMI were associated with diastolic blood pressure (DBP) and mean arterial pressure (MAP). Moreover, after eight years, baseline BAI and

BMI were associated with changes (Δ) in systolic BP, MAP, and pulse pressure, while only BMI was positively related to ΔDBP. They concluded that BAI and BMI were significant predictors of risk of HTN and changes in BP after an 8-years follow-up [96].

CONICITY INDEX (C-INDEX)

Conicity index (C-index) is calculated according to WC, weight, and height. In 1991, Valdez firstly described it as a simple model-based index of abdominal adiposity [97]. The C-index has been used to investigate the prediction of long-term cardiometabolic risk among middle-aged males and females and demonstrated good clinical discriminatory value for long-term cardiometabolic risk. Abulmeaty and colleagues found that the VAI, C-index, and mid-arm muscular areas were the best discriminators of the long-term cardiometabolic risk in men and not in women. They concluded that long-term cardiometabolic risk could be predicted using simple anthropometric and central obesity indices, and these discriminators were not the same in Saudi men and women [98]. Kommuri and colleagues explored the associations between various anthropometric and subclinical atherosclerosis markers in a longitudinal cohort study in 6,814 participants. They concluded that C-index was a less consistent marker associated with various subclinical atherosclerosis markers than other anthropometric measures [30]. However, in 2015, another study showed that C-index (AUC: 0.67– 0.76) had the highest discriminatory accuracy to predict 10-year CV events compared with WC (AUC: 0.57–0.59), WHtR (AUC: 0.62–0.65), and AVI (AUC, 0.57–0.59). They concluded that C-index and WHR had a more discriminatory accuracy for 10-year CV events than the other obesity indices [99]. In 2018, Zhang and colleagues conducted a study to compare six anthropometric indices' predictive ability to identify metabolic syndrome (MetS) and determine their optimal cut-off points among 59,029 Chinese adults.

They concluded that C-index was not a superior predictor for MetS compared with BMI, WC, WHtR, and body roundness index (BRI) [100]. In 2019, 4 studies were conducted to investigate the capacity of different anthropometric measures, especially C-index related to diabetes, cardiometabolic risks, and MetS. All four studies concluded that C-index was a useful parameter associated with diabetes, cardiometabolic risks, and MetS. However, it was not superior above the conventional anthropometric parameters [101, 102, 103, 104].

CONCLUSION

Although obesity is a significant risk factor for cardiovascular events, some studies showed that obesity could decrease mortality. This obesity paradox occurred in some chronic conditions, with obese individuals presenting with a survival advantage over their counterparts. BMI has several limitations because it does not accurately differentiate different body composition components. Assessing fat and its distribution in different body regions was of great significance in predicting cardiovascular risk factors. The current non-invasive techniques comprising many anthropometric measurements and indices play a critical role in detecting, evaluating, and determining body adiposity, body fatness, and distribution. Different adiposity indices and anthropometric measures showed varying degrees of association with body fat proportions and cardiovascular risk factors. However, to determine the better predictor of obesity jeopardy associated with cardiometabolic risks, the well designed, randomized controlled trial was needed. Base on the extensive observational and cross-sectional studies, WHHtR, WHtR, and SADHtR, seem to be the better anthropometric parameters to predict CV risks among the obesity population. While WTR, BAI, and C-index do not demonstrate superiority over BMI.

REFERENCES

[1] Grundy, Scott M. "Metabolic Complications of Obesity." *Endocrine* 13, no. 2 (2000): 155-65. doi:10.1385/endo:13:2:155.

[2] Vettor, Roberto, and Scilla Conci. "Obesity Pathogenesis." *Endocrinology Obesity*, 2019, 89-108. doi:10.1007/978-3-319-46933-1_14.

[3] Engin, Atilla. "The Definition and Prevalence of Obesity and Metabolic Syndrome." *Obesity and Lipotoxicity Advances in Experimental Medicine and Biology*, 2017, 1-17. doi:10.1007/978-3-319-48382-5_1.

[4] Nimptsch, Katharina, Stefan Konigorski, and Tobias Pischon. "Diagnosis of Obesity and Use of Obesity Biomarkers in Science and Clinical Medicine." *Metabolism* 92 (2019): 61-70. doi:10.1016/j.metabol.2018.12.006.

[5] "Overweight and Obesity." 2020. doi:10.1787/a47d0cd2-en.

[6] Iacobellis, Gianluca. "Introduction: Redefinition of the Relationship between Obesity and the Cardiovascular System." *Obesity and Cardiovascular Disease*, 2009, 1-4. doi:10.1093/med/9780199549320.003.0001.

[7] Guerra, Alberto Francisco Rubio. "Association between Epicardial Fat, Metabolic Syndrome and Obesity." *Journal of Diabetes and Obesity* 2, no. 4 (2015): 1-3. doi:10.15436/2376-0494.15.034.

[8] "Mortality from Cardiovascular Disease." 2020. doi:10.1787/cce902d8-en.

[9] Carlson, Scott H., and J. Michael Wyss. "Mechanisms Underlying Hypertension and Obesity." *Hypertension* 57, no. 3 (2011): 375-76. doi:10.1161/hypertensionaha.110.161729.

[10] Parmar, Mihir Y. "Obesity and Type 2 Diabetes Mellitus." *Integrative Obesity and Diabetes* 4, no. 4 (2018). doi:10.15761/iod.1000217.

[11] Kotsis, Vasilios, Christina Antza, Giannis Doundoulakis, and Stella Stabouli. "Obesity, Hypertension, and Dyslipidemia." *Endocrinology Obesity*, 2019, 227-41. doi:10.1007/978-3-319-46933-1_22.

[12] Jayawardena, Ranil, Priyanga Ranasinghe, Thilina Ranathunga, Yasith Mathangasinghe, Sudharshani Wasalathanththri, and Andrew P. Hills. "Novel Anthropometric Parameters to Define Obesity and Obesity-related Disease in Adults: A Systematic Review." *Nutrition Reviews* 78, no. 6 (2019): 498-513. doi:10.1093/nutrit/nuz078.

[13] Gruberg, Luis, Neil J. Weissman, Ron Waksman, Shmuel Fuchs, Regina Deible, Ellen E. Pinnow, Lanja M. Ahmed, Kenneth M. Kent, Augusto D. Pichard, William O. Suddath, Lowell F. Satler, and Joseph Lindsay. "The Impact of Obesity on the Short-term And long-term Outcomes after Percutaneous Coronary Intervention: The Obesity Paradox?" *Journal of the American College of Cardiology* 39, no. 4 (2002): 578-84. doi:10.1016/s0735-1097(01)01802-2.

[14] Carbone, Salvatore, Justin M. Canada, Hayley E. Billingsley, Mohammad S. Siddiqui, Andrew Elagizi, and Carl J. Lavie. "Obesity Paradox in Cardiovascular Disease: Where Do We Stand?" *Vascular Health and Risk Management* Volume 15 (2019): 89-100. doi:10.2147/vhrm.s168946.

[15] Xia, Jonathan Y., Donald M. Lloyd-Jones, and Sadiya S. Khan. "Association of Body Mass Index with Mortality in Cardiovascular Disease: New Insights into the Obesity Paradox from Multiple Perspectives." *Trends in Cardiovascular Medicine* 29, no. 4 (2019): 220-25. doi:10.1016/j.tcm.2018.08.006.

[16] Flegal, Katherine M., Brian K. Kit, Heather Orpana, and Barry I. Graubard. 2013. "Association of All-Cause Mortality with Overweight and Obesity Using Standard Body Mass Index Categories." *JAMA* 309 (1): 71. https://doi.org/10.1001/jama.2012.113905.

[17] Zhang, Jufen, Aine Begley, Ruth Jackson, Michael Harrison, Pierpaolo Pellicori, Andrew L. Clark, and John G. F. Cleland. "Body Mass Index and All-Cause Mortality in Heart Failure Patients with Normal and Reduced Ventricular Ejection Fraction: a Dose-Response Meta-Analysis." *Clinical Research in Cardiology* 108, no. 2 (2018): 119–32. https://doi.org/ 10.1007/ s00392-018-1302-7.

[18] Prado, Carla M., M. Cristina Gonzalez, and Steven B. Heymsfield. 2015. "Body Composition Phenotypes and Obesity Paradox." *Current Opinion in Clinical Nutrition and Metabolic Care* 18 (6): 535–51. https://doi.org/10.1097/mco. 0000000000000216.

[19] Heymsfield, Steven B., and William T. Cefalu. 2013. "Does Body Mass Index Adequately Convey a Patient's Mortality Risk?" *JAMA* 309 (1): 87. https://doi.org/ 10.1001/jama.2012.185445.

[20] Romero-Corral, A., V. K. Somers, J. Sierra-Johnson, R. J. Thomas, M. L. Collazo-Clavell, J. Korinek, T. G. Allison, J. A. Batsis, F. H. Sert-Kuniyoshi, and F. Lopez-Jimenez. "Accuracy of Body Mass Index in Diagnosing Obesity in the Adult General Population." *International Journal of Obesity* 32, no. 6 (2008): 959-66. doi:10.1038/ijo.2008.11.

[21] Rothman, K. J. "BMI-related Errors in the Measurement of Obesity." *International Journal of Obesity* 32, no. S3 (2008). doi:10.1038/ijo. 2008.87.

[22] Leowattana, Wattana. "Obesity and Acute Cardiovascular Events." *European Journal of Preventive Cardiology* 25, no. 6 (2018): 618-20. doi:10.1177/2047487318758361.

[23] Dwivedi, Alok Kumar, Pallavi Dubey, David P. Cistola, and Sireesha Y. Reddy. "Association between Obesity and Cardiovascular Outcomes: Updated Evidence from Meta-analysis Studies." *Current Cardiology Reports* 22, no. 4 (2020). doi:10.1007/s11886-020-1273-y.

[24] Song, X., P. Jousilahti, C. D. A. Stehouwer, S. Söderberg, A. Onat, T. Laatikainen, J. S. Yudkin, R. Dankner, R. Morris, J. Tuomilehto, and Q. Qiao. "Comparison of Various Surrogate Obesity Indicators as Predictors of Cardiovascular Mortality in Four European Populations." *European Journal of Clinical Nutrition* 67, no. 12 (2013): 1298-302. doi:10.1038/ejcn.2013.203.

[25] Hsieh, Shiun Dong, and Hideyo Yoshinaga. 1995. "Waist/Height Ratio as A Simple and Useful Predictor of Coronary Heart Disease Risk Factors in Women." *Internal Medicine* 34 (12): 1147–52. https://doi.org/10.2169/ internalmedicine.34. 1147.

[26] Ononamadu, Chimaobi James, Chinwe Nonyelum Ezekwesili, Onyemaechi Faith Onyeukwu, Uchenna Francis Umeoguaju, Obiajulu Christian Ezeigwe, and Godwin Okwudiri Ihegboro. 2017. "Comparative Analysis of Anthropometric Indices of Obesity as Correlates and Potential Predictors of Risk for Hypertension and Prehypertension in a Population in Nigeria." *Cardiovascular Journal of Africa* 28 (2): 92–99. https://doi.org/ 10.5830/cvja-2016-061.

[27] Li, Chaoyang, Earl S. Ford, Guixiang Zhao, Henry S. Kahn, and Ali H. Mokdad. 2010. "Waist-to-Thigh Ratio and Diabetes among US Adults: The Third National Health and Nutrition Examination Survey." *Diabetes Research and Clinical Practice* 89 (1): 79–87. https://doi.org/ 10.1016/j.diabres.2010.02.014.

[28] Carlsson, A. C., U. Risérus, G. Engström, J. Ärnlöv, O. Melander, K. Leander, B. Gigante, M. L. Hellénius, and U. de Faire. 2013. "Novel and Established Anthropometric Measures and the Prediction of Incident Cardiovascular Disease: A Cohort Study." *International Journal of Obesity* 37 (12): 1579–85. https://doi.org/10.1038/ijo.2013.46.

[29] Fu, Shihui, Leiming Luo, Ping Ye, Yuan Liu, Yongyi Bai, Jie Bai, and Bing Zhu. 2014. "The Abilities of New Anthropometric Indices in Identifying Cardiometabolic Abnormalities, and Influence of Residence Area and Lifestyle on These Anthropometric Indices in a Chinese Community-Dwelling Population." *Clinical Interventions in Aging*, January, 179. https://doi.org/10.2147/cia.s54240.

[30] Kommuri, Naga V. A., Sandip K. Zalawadiya, Vikas Veeranna, Sri Lakshmi S. Kollepara, Krithi Ramesh, Alexandros Briasoulis, and Luis Afonso. 2015. "Association between Various Anthropometric Measures of Obesity and Markers of Subclinical Atherosclerosis." *Expert Review of Cardiovascular Therapy* 14 (1): 127–35. https://doi.org/10.1586/ 14779072.2016.1118346.

[31] Lavie, Carl J., Alban De Schutter, Parham Parto, Eiman Jahangir, Peter Kokkinos, Francisco B. Ortega, Ross Arena, and Richard V. Milani. 2016. "Obesity and Prevalence of Cardiovascular Diseases and Prognosis—The Obesity Paradox Updated." *Progress in*

Cardiovascular Diseases 58 (5): 537–47. https://doi.org/ 10.1016/ j.pcad. 2016.01.008.

[32] Nakamura, Kazuto, José J. Fuster, and Kenneth Walsh. 2014. "Adipokines: A Link between Obesity and Cardiovascular Disease." *Journal of Cardiology* 63 (4): 250–59. https://doi.org/10.1016/ j.jjcc.2013.11.006.

[33] Kim, Jung A., and Kyung Mook Choi. 2020. "Newly Discovered Adipokines: Pathophysiological Link between Obesity and Cardiometabolic Disorders." *Frontiers in Physiology* 11 (September). https://doi.org/10.3389/fphys.2020.568800.

[34] Cinti, Saverio, Grant Mitchell, Giorgio Barbatelli, Incoronata Murano, Enzo Ceresi, Emanuela Faloia, Shupei Wang, Melanie Fortier, Andrew S. Greenberg, and Martin S. Obin. 2005. "Adipocyte Death Defines Macrophage Localization and Function in Adipose Tissue of Obese Mice and Humans." *Journal of Lipid Research* 46 (11): 2347–55. https://doi.org/10.1194/jlr.m500294-jlr200.

[35] Zhang, John, and Pronyuk KHO. 2015. "Adiponectin, Resistin, and Leptin: Possible Markers of Metabolic Syndrome." *Endocrinology & Metabolic Syndrome* 04 (04). https://doi.org/10.4172/2161-1017.100 0212.

[36] Ginsberg, Henry N., Yuan-Li Zhang, and Antonio Hernandez-Ono. 2006. "Metabolic Syndrome: Focus on Dyslipidemia." *Obesity* 14 (2S): 41S-49S. https://doi.org/ 10.1038/oby.2006.281.

[37] Lavie, Carl J., Paul A. McAuley, Timothy S. Church, Richard V. Milani, and Steven N. Blair. 2014. "Obesity and Cardiovascular Diseases." *Journal of the American College of Cardiology* 63 (14): 1345–54. https://doi.org/10.1016/j.jacc.2014.01.022.

[38] Gelber, R., J. Gaziano, J. Manson, J. Buring, and H. Sesso. 2007. "A Prospective Study of Body Mass Index and the Risk of Developing Hypertension in Men." *American Journal of Hypertension* 20 (4): 370–77. https://doi.org/10.1016/j.amjhyper. 2006. 10.011.

[39] Hall, John E., Jussara M. do Carmo, Alexandre A. da Silva, and John D. Dubinion. 2012. "Pathophysiology of Obesity and Hypertension."

Journal of Hypertension 30 (September): e114–15. https://doi.org/ 10.1097/01.hjh. 0000420237.69136.84.

[40] Kandilova, V. N. 2020. "Cardiac and Vascular Remodeling in Arterial Hypertension: The Role of Concomitant Obesity." *The Clinician* 14 (1–2): 62–72. https://doi.org/ 10.17650/1818-8338-2020-14-1-2-62-72.

[41] Litwin, Sheldon E. 2010. "Cardiac Remodeling in Obesity." *JACC: Cardiovascular Imaging* 3 (3): 275–77. https://doi.org/10.1016/ j.jcmg. 2009.12.004.

[42] Neeland, Ian J., Sachin Gupta, Colby R. Ayers, Aslan T. Turer, J. Eduardo Rame, Sandeep R. Das, Jarett D. Berry, et al. 2013. "Relation of Regional Fat Distribution to Left Ventricular Structure and Function." *Circulation: Cardiovascular Imaging* 6 (5): 800–807. https://doi.org/10.1161/ circimaging.113.000532.

[43] Moore, L. L., A. J. Visioni, and M. M. Qureshi. 2005. "Weight Loss in Overweight Adults and the Long-Term Risk of Hypertension: The Framingham Study." *ACC Current Journal Review* 14 (9): 6–7. https://doi.org/10.1016/j.accreview.2005.08.190.

[44] Weiss, Ram, Andrew A. Bremer, and Robert H. Lustig. 2013. "What Is Metabolic Syndrome, and Why Are Children Getting It?" *Annals of the New York Academy of Sciences* 1281 (1): 123–40. https://doi.org/10.1111/nyas.12030.

[45] Alberti, K. George M. M., Paul Zimmet, and Jonathan Shaw. 2005. "The Metabolic Syndrome—a New Worldwide Definition." *The Lancet* 366 (9491): 1059–62. https://doi.org/10.1016/s0140-6736(05)67402-8.

[46] Grundy, Scott M. 2008. "Metabolic Syndrome Pandemic." *Arteriosclerosis, Thrombosis, and Vascular Biology* 28 (4): 629–36. https://doi.org/10.1161/atvbaha. 107.151092.

[47] Amin, Mohammad Nurul, Md. Saddam Hussain, Md. Shahid Sarwar, Md. Mizanur Rahman Moghal, Abhijit Das, Mohammad Zahid Hossain, Jakir Ahmed Chowdhury, Md. Shalahuddin Millat, and Mohammad Safiqul Islam. 2019. "How the Association between Obesity and Inflammation May Lead to Insulin Resistance and

Cancer." *Diabetes & Metabolic Syndrome: Clinical Research & Reviews* 13 (2): 1213–24. https://doi.org/10.1016/j.dsx.2019.01.041.

[48] Zafar, Uzma, Saba Khaliq, Hafiz Usman Ahmad, Sobia Manzoor, and Khalid P. Lone. 2018. "Metabolic Syndrome: An Update on Diagnostic Criteria, Pathogenesis, and Genetic Links." *Hormones (Athens, Greece)* 17 (3): 299–313. https://doi.org/10.1007/ s42000-018-0051-3.

[49] Katzmarzyk, P. T., T. S. Church, I. Janssen, R. Ross, and S. N. Blair. 2005. "Metabolic Syndrome, Obesity, and Mortality: Impact of Cardiorespiratory Fitness." *Diabetes Care* 28 (2): 391–97. https://doi.org/10.2337/diacare. 28.2.391.

[50] Isomaa, B., P. Almgren, T. Tuomi, B. Forsen, K. Lahti, M. Nissen, M.-R. Taskinen, and L. Groop. 2001. "Cardiovascular Morbidity and Mortality Associated With the Metabolic Syndrome." *Diabetes Care* 24 (4): 683–89. https://doi.org/10.2337/diacare. 24.4.683.

[51] Calori, Giliola, Guido Lattuada, Lorenzo Piemonti, Maria Paola Garancini, Francesca Ragogna, Marco Villa, Salvatore Mannino, et al. 2011. "Prevalence, Metabolic Features, and Prognosis of Metabolically Healthy Obese Italian Individuals." *Diabetes Care* 34 (1): 210–215. https://doi.org/10.2337/dc10-0665.

[52] Fan, Jingyao, Yiqing Song, Yu Chen, Rutai Hui, and Weili Zhang. 2013. "Combined Effect of Obesity and Cardio-Metabolic Abnormality on the Risk of Cardiovascular Disease: A Meta-Analysis of Prospective Cohort Studies." *International Journal of Cardiology* 168 (5): 4761–68. https://doi.org/10.1016/j.ijcard.2013. 07.230.

[53] Ortega, Francisco B., Cristina Cadenas-Sánchez, Xuemei Sui, Steven N. Blair, and Carl J. Lavie. 2015. "Role of Fitness in the Metabolically Healthy but Obese Phenotype: A Review and Update." *Progress in Cardiovascular Diseases* 58 (1): 76–86. https://doi.org/10. 1016/j.pcad.2015.05.001.

[54] Li, Jian, and Johannes Siegrist. 2012. "Physical Activity and Risk of Cardiovascular Disease—A Meta-Analysis of Prospective Cohort Studies." *International Journal of Environmental Research and*

Public Health 9 (2): 391–407. https://doi.org/10.3390/ijerph9020391.

[55] Parto, Parham, Carl J. Lavie, Damon Swift, and Xuemei Sui. 2015. "The Role of Cardiorespiratory Fitness on Plasma Lipid Levels." *Expert Review of Cardiovascular Therapy* 13 (11): 1177–83. https://doi.org/10.1586/14779072.2015.1092384.

[56] Fernandez, Celine, Marianne Sandin, Julio L. Sampaio, Peter Almgren, Krzysztof Narkiewicz, Michal Hoffmann, Thomas Hedner, et al. 2013. "Plasma Lipid Composition and Risk of Developing Cardiovascular Disease." Edited by Stefan Kiechl. *PLoS ONE* 8 (8): e71846. https://doi.org/10.1371/journal.pone.0071846.

[57] Park, Yong-Moon Mark, Xuemei Sui, Junxiu Liu, Haiming Zhou, Peter F. Kokkinos, Carl J. Lavie, James W. Hardin, and Steven N. Blair. 2015. "The Effect of Cardiorespiratory Fitness on Age-Related Lipids and Lipoproteins." *Journal of the American College of Cardiology* 65 (19): 2091–2100. https://doi.org/10.1016/j.jacc.2015.03.517.

[58] Cullen, Paul. 2000. "Evidence That Triglycerides Are an Independent Coronary Heart Disease Risk Factor." *The American Journal of Cardiology* 86 (9): 943–49. https://doi.org/10.1016/s0002-9149(00)01127-9.

[59] Klop, Boudewijn, Jan Elte, and Manuel Cabezas. 2013. "Dyslipidemia in Obesity: Mechanisms and Potential Targets." *Nutrients* 5 (4): 1218–40. https://doi.org/10.3390/ nu5041218.

[60] Lin, Chenchen, Tarja Rajalahti, Svein Are Mjøs, and Olav Martin Kvalheim. 2015. "Predictive Associations between Serum Fatty Acids and Lipoproteins in Healthy Non-Obese Norwegians: Implications for Cardiovascular Health." *Metabolomics* 12 (1). https://doi.org/10.1007/s11306-015-0886-4.

[61] Mc Loughlin, Santiago, and Gaston A. Rodriguez-Granillo. 2012. "HDL-C Levels and Cardiovascular Disease: More Is Not Always Better!" *Recent Patents on Cardiovascular Drug Discovery* 7 (2): 121–33. https://doi.org/10.2174/1574890128 01227283.

[62] Arner, Peter, and Mikael Rydén. 2015. "Fatty Acids, Obesity and Insulin Resistance." *Obesity Facts* 8 (2): 147–55. https://doi.org/10.1159/000381224.

[63] Lottenberg, Ana Maria, Milessa da Silva Afonso, Maria Silvia Ferrari Lavrador, Roberta Marcondes Machado, and Edna Regina Nakandakare. 2012. "The Role of Dietary Fatty Acids in the Pathology of Metabolic Syndrome." *The Journal of Nutritional Biochemistry* 23 (9): 1027–40. https://doi.org/10.1016/j.jnutbio. 2012.03.004.

[64] Litwin, Sheldon E. 2010. "Cardiac Remodeling in Obesity." *JACC: Cardiovascular Imaging* 3 (3): 275–77. https://doi.org/10.1016/j.jcmg.2009.12.004.

[65] Kenchaiah, Satish, Jane C. Evans, Daniel Levy, Peter W.F. Wilson, Emelia J. Benjamin, Martin G. Larson, William B. Kannel, and Ramachandran S. Vasan. 2002. "Obesity and the Risk of Heart Failure." *New England Journal of Medicine* 347 (5): 305–13. https://doi.org/10.1056/nejmoa020245.

[66] Kenchaiah, Satish, Howard D. Sesso, and J. Michael Gaziano. 2009. "Body Mass Index and Vigorous Physical Activity and the Risk of Heart Failure Among Men." *Circulation* 119 (1): 44–52. https://doi.org/10.1161/circulationaha.108.807289.

[67] Hu, Gang, Pekka Jousilahti, Riitta Antikainen, Peter T. Katzmarzyk, and Jaakko Tuomilehto. 2010. "Joint Effects of Physical Activity, Body Mass Index, Waist Circumference, and Waist-to-Hip Ratio on the Risk of Heart Failure." *Circulation* 121 (2): 237–44. https://doi.org/10.1161/circulationaha.109.887893.

[68] Levitan, Emily B., Amy Z. Yang, Alicja Wolk, and Murray A. Mittleman. 2009. "Adiposity and Incidence of Heart Failure Hospitalization and Mortality." Circulation: *Heart Failure* 2 (3): 202–8. https://doi.org/10.1161/circheartfailure.108.794099.

[69] Savji, Nazir, Wouter C. Meijers, Traci M. Bartz, Vijeta Bhambhani, Mary Cushman, Matthew Nayor, Jorge R. Kizer, et al. 2018. "The Association of Obesity and Cardiometabolic Traits With Incident

HFpEF and HFrEF." *JACC: Heart Failure* 6 (8): 701–9. https://doi.org/10.1016/j.jchf.2018.05.018.

[70] Wang, Thomas J. 2004. "Obesity and the Risk of New-Onset Atrial Fibrillation." *JAMA* 292 (20): 2471. https://doi.org/10.1001/jama.292.20.2471.

[71] Frost, Lars, Emelia J. Benjamin, Morten Fenger-Grøn, Asger Pedersen, Anne Tjønneland, and Kim Overvad. 2014. "Body Fat, Body Fat Distribution, Lean Body Mass and Atrial Fibrillation and Flutter. A Danish Cohort Study." *Obesity* 22 (6): 1546–52. https://doi.org/10.1002/oby.20706.

[72] Schmidt, Morten, Hans Erik Bøtker, Lars Pedersen, and Henrik Toft Sørensen. 2014. "Comparison of the Frequency of Atrial Fibrillation in Young Obese Versus Young Nonobese Men Undergoing Examination for Fitness for Military Service." *The American Journal of Cardiology* 113 (5): 822–26. https://doi.org/10.1016/j.amjcard.2013.11.037.

[73] Özcan, Kazım Serhan, Barış Güngör, Servet Altay, Damirbek Osmonov, Ahmet Ekmekçi, Fatma Özpamuk, Tuğba Kemaloğlu, Aydın Yıldırım, Gülşah Tayyareci, and İzzet Erdinler. 2014. "Increased Level of Resistin Predicts Development of Atrial Fibrillation." *Journal of Cardiology* 63 (4): 308–12. https://doi.org/10.1016/j.jjcc. 2013.10.008.

[74] Sandhu, Roopinder K., David Conen, Usha B. Tedrow, Kathryn C. Fitzgerald, Aruna D. Pradhan, Paul M Ridker, Robert J. Glynn, and Christine M. Albert. 2014. "Predisposing Factors Associated With Development of Persistent Compared With Paroxysmal Atrial Fibrillation." *Journal of the American Heart Association* 3 (3). https://doi.org/10.1161/jaha.114.000916.

[75] Thacker, Evan L., Barbara McKnight, Bruce M. Psaty, W. T. Longstreth, Sascha Dublin, Paul N. Jensen, Katherine M. Newton, Nicholas L. Smith, David S. Siscovick, and Susan R. Heckbert. 2012. "Association of Body Mass Index, Diabetes, Hypertension, and Blood Pressure Levels with Risk of Permanent Atrial Fibrillation."

Journal of General Internal Medicine 28 (2): 247–53. https://doi.org/10.1007/s11606-012-2220-4.

[76] Guijian, Liu, Yan Jinchuan, Du Rongzeng, Qian Jun, Wu Jun, and Zhu Wenqing. 2013. "Impact of Body Mass Index on Atrial Fibrillation Recurrence: A Meta-Analysis of Observational Studies." *Pacing and Clinical Electrophysiology* 36 (6): 748–56. https://doi.org/10.1111/pace.12106.

[77] Pouwels, Sjaak, Besir Topal, Mireille T. Knook, Alper Celik, Magnus Sundbom, Rui Ribeiro, Chetan Parmar, and Surendra Ugale. 2019. "Interaction of Obesity and Atrial Fibrillation: An Overview of Pathophysiology and Clinical Management." *Expert Review of Cardiovascular Therapy* 17 (3): 209–23. https://doi.org/10.1080/14779072.2019.1581064.

[78] Fu, Shihui, Leiming Luo, Ping Ye, Yuan Liu, Yongyi Bai, Jie Bai, and Bing Zhu. 2014. "The Abilities of New Anthropometric Indices in Identifying Cardiometabolic Abnormalities, and Influence of Residence Area and Lifestyle on These Anthropometric Indices in a Chinese Community-Dwelling Population." *Clinical Interventions in Aging*, January, 179. https://doi.org/10.2147/cia.s54240.

[79] Carlsson, A.C., U. Riserus, J. Ärnlöv, Y. Borné, K. Leander, B. Gigante, M.-L. Hellénius, M. Bottai, and U. de Faire. 2014. "Prediction of Cardiovascular Disease by Abdominal Obesity Measures Is Dependent on Body Weight and Sex – Results from Two Community Based Cohort Studies." *Nutrition, Metabolism and Cardiovascular Diseases* 24 (8): 891–99. https://doi.org/10.1016/j.numecd.2014.02.001.

[80] Hardy, Dale S., Devita T. Stallings, Jane T. Garvin, Hongyan Xu, and Susan B. Racette. 2017. "Best Anthropometric Discriminators of Incident Type 2 Diabetes among White and Black Adults: A Longitudinal ARIC Study." Edited by David Meyre. *PLOS ONE* 12 (1): e0168282. https://doi.org/10.1371/journal.pone.0168282.

[81] Browning, Lucy M., Shiun Dong Hsieh, and Margaret Ashwell. 2010. "A Systematic Review of Waist-to-Height Ratio as a Screening Tool for the Prediction of Cardiovascular Disease and Diabetes: 0·5 Could Be a Suitable Global Boundary Value." *Nutrition Research Reviews* 23 (2): 247–69. https://doi.org/10.1017/ s09544224100 00144.

[82] Ashwell, M., P. Gunn, and S. Gibson. 2011. "Waist-to-Height Ratio Is a Better Screening Tool than Waist Circumference and BMI for Adult Cardiometabolic Risk Factors: Systematic Review and Meta-Analysis." *Obesity Reviews* 13 (3): 275–86. https://doi.org/10.1111/ j.1467-789x.2011.00952.x.

[83] Corrêa, Márcia Mara, Elaine Thumé, Elizabete Regina Araújo De Oliveira, and Elaine Tomasi. 2016. "Performance of the Waist-to-Height Ratio in Identifying Obesity and Predicting Non-Communicable Diseases in the Elderly Population: A Systematic Literature Review." *Archives of Gerontology and Geriatrics* 65 (July): 174–82. https://doi.org/10.1016/j.archger.2016.03.021.

[84] Rangel-Baltazar, Eduardo, Lucia Cuevas-Nasu, Teresa Shamah-Levy, Sonia Rodríguez-Ramírez, Ignacio Méndez-Gómez-Humarán, and Juan A Rivera. 2019. "Association between High Waist-to-Height Ratio and Cardiovascular Risk among Adults Sampled by the 2016 Half-Way National Health and Nutrition Survey in Mexico (ENSANUT MC 2016)." *Nutrients* 11 (6): 1402. https://doi.org/ 10.3390/nu11061402.

[85] Lo, Kenneth, Yu-Qing Huang, Geng Shen, Jia-Yi Huang, Lin Liu, Yu-Ling Yu, Chao-Lei Chen, and Ying Qing Feng. 2020. "Effects of Waist to Height Ratio, Waist Circumference, Body Mass Index on the Risk of Chronic Diseases, All-Cause, Cardiovascular and Cancer Mortality." *Postgraduate Medical Journal*, May, postgradmedj-2020-137542. https://doi.org/10.1136/postgradmedj-2020-137542.

[86] Fay, Roger A., Philip L. Dey, Christopher M.J. Saadie, Janice A. Buhl, and Val J. Gebski. 1991. "Ponderal Index: A Better Definition of the 'At Risk' Group With Intrauterine Growth Problems than Birth-Weight for Gestational Age in Term Infants." *The Australian and New Zealand Journal of Obstetrics and Gynaecology* 31 (1): 17–19. https://doi.org/10.1111/j.1479-828x.1991.tb02755.x.

[87] Ononamadu, Chimaobi James, Chinwe Nonyelum Ezekwesili, Onyemaechi Faith Onyeukwu, Uchenna Francis Umeoguaju, Obiajulu Christian Ezeigwe, and Godwin Okwudiri Ihegboro. 2017. "Comparative Analysis of Anthropometric Indices of Obesity as Correlates and Potential Predictors of Risk for Hypertension and Prehypertension in a Population in Nigeria." *Cardiovascular Journal of Africa* 28 (2): 92–99. https://doi.org/10.5830/cvja-2016-061.

[88] Lu, Bing, Jing Zhou, Molly E. Waring, Donna R. Parker, and Charles B. Eaton. 2010. "Abdominal Obesity and Peripheral Vascular Disease in Men and Women: A Comparison of Waist-to-Thigh Ratio and Waist Circumference as Measures of Abdominal Obesity." *Atherosclerosis* 208 (1): 253–57. https://doi.org/10.1016/j.atherosclerosis.2009.06.027.

[89] Beraldo, Rebeca A, Gabriela C Meliscki, Bruna R Silva, Anderson M Navarro, Valdes R Bollela, André Schmidt, and Maria C Foss-Freitas. 2018. "Anthropometric Measures of Central Adiposity Are Highly Concordant with Predictors of Cardiovascular Disease Risk in HIV Patients." *The American Journal of Clinical Nutrition* 107 (6): 883–93. https://doi.org/10.1093/ajcn/nqy049.

[90] Kumlin, L., L. Dimberg, and P. Marin. 1997. "Ratio of Abdominal Sagittal Diameter to Height Is Strong Indicator of Coronary Risk." *BMJ* 314 (7083): 830–830. https://doi.org/10.1136/bmj.314.7083.830.

[91] Bertin, E, C Marcus, J-C Ruiz, J-P Eschard, and M Leutenegger. 2000. "Measurement of Visceral Adipose Tissue by DXA Combined with Anthropometry in Obese Humans." *International Journal of Obesity* 24 (3): 263–70. https://doi.org/10.1038/ sj.ijo.0801121.

[92] Kahn, Henry S., and Yiling J. Cheng. 2018. "Comparison of Adiposity Indicators Associated with Fasting-State Insulinemia, Triglyceridemia, and Related Risk Biomarkers in a Nationally Representative, Adult Population." *Diabetes Research and Clinical Practice* 136 (February): 7–15. https://doi.org/10.1016/j.diabres. 2017.11. 019.

[93] Bergman, Richard N., Darko Stefanovski, Thomas A. Buchanan, Anne E. Sumner, James C. Reynolds, Nancy G. Sebring, Anny H. Xiang, and Richard M. Watanabe. 2011. "A Better Index of Body Adiposity." *Obesity* 19 (5): 1083–89. https://doi.org/ 10.1038/oby. 2011.38.

[94] Lam, Benjamin Chih Chiang, Gerald Choon Huat Koh, Cynthia Chen, Michael Tack Keong Wong, and Stephen J. Fallows. 2015. "Comparison of Body Mass Index (BMI), Body Adiposity Index (BAI), Waist Circumference (WC), Waist-To-Hip Ratio (WHR) and Waist-To-Height Ratio (WHtR) as Predictors of Cardiovascular Disease Risk Factors in an Adult Population in Singapore." Edited by Pedro Tauler. *PLOS ONE* 10 (4): e0122985. https://doi.org/10. 1371/journal.pone.0122985.

[95] Belarmino, Giliane, Lilian Mika Horie, Priscila Campos Sala, Raquel S. Torrinhas, Steven B. Heymsfield, and Dan L. Waitzberg. 2015. "Body Adiposity Index Performance in Estimating Body Fat in a Sample of Severely Obese Brazilian Patients." *Nutrition Journal* 14 (1). https://doi.org/10.1186/s12937-015-0119-8.

[96] D'Elia, L., M. Manfredi, P. Sabino, P. Strazzullo, and F. Galletti. 2016. "The Olivetti Heart Study: Predictive Value of a New Adiposity Index on Risk of Hypertension, Blood Pressure, and Subclinical Organ Damage." *Nutrition, Metabolism and Cardiovascular Diseases* 26 (7): 630–36. https://doi.org/10.1016/ j.numecd.2016.03. 009.

[97] Valdez, R. 1991. "A Simple Model-Based Index of Abdominal Adiposity." *Journal of Clinical Epidemiology* 44 (9): 955–56. https://doi.org/10.1016/0895-4356(91)90059-i.

[98] Abulmeaty, Mahmoud, Ali Almajwal, Najwa Almadani, Mona Aldosari, Ahmed Alnajim, Saeed Ali, Heba Hassan, and Hany Elkatawy. 2017. "Anthropometric and Central Obesity Indices as Predictors of Long-Term Cardiometabolic Risk among Saudi Young and Middle-Aged Men and Women." *Saudi Medical Journal* 38 (4): 372–80. https://doi.org/10.15537/smj.2017.4.18758.

[99] Motamed, Nima, Dhaya Perumal, Farhad Zamani, Hossein Ashrafi, Majid Haghjoo, F.S. Saeedian, Mansooreh Maadi, Haleh Akhavan-Niaki, Behnam Rabiee, and Mohsen Asouri. 2015. "Conicity Index and Waist-to-Hip Ratio Are Superior Obesity Indices in Predicting 10-Year Cardiovascular Risk Among Men and Women." *Clinical Cardiology* 38 (9): 527–34. https://doi.org/10.1002/clc.22437.

[100] Zhang, Jia, Wenhua Zhu, Lifeng Qiu, Lijuan Huang, and Lizheng Fang. 2018. "Sex- and Age-Specific Optimal Anthropometric Indices as Screening Tools for Metabolic Syndrome in Chinese Adults." *International Journal of Endocrinology* 2018 (September): 1–16. https://doi.org/10.1155/2018/1067603.

[101] Wang, Z., S. He, and X. Chen. 2019. "Capacity of Different Anthropometric Measures to Predict Diabetes in a Chinese Population in Southwest China: A 15-year Prospective Study." *Diabetic Medicine* 36 (10): 1261–67. https://doi.org/10.1111/dme.14055.

[102] Ramírez-Vélez, Robinson, Miguel Ángel Pérez-Sousa, Mikel Izquierdo, Carlos A. Cano-Gutierrez, Emilio González-Jiménez, Jacqueline Schmidt-RioValle, Katherine González-Ruíz, and María Correa-Rodríguez. 2019. "Validation of Surrogate Anthropometric Indices in Older Adults: What Is the Best Indicator of High Cardiometabolic Risk Factor Clustering?" *Nutrients* 11 (8): 1701. https://doi.org/ 10.3390/nu11081701.

[103] Quaye, Lawrence, William Kwame Boakye Ansah Owiredu, Nafiu Amidu, Peter Paul Mwinsanga Dapare, and Yussif Adams. 2019. "Comparative Abilities of Body Mass Index, Waist Circumference, Abdominal Volume Index, Body Adiposity Index, and Conicity Index as Predictive Screening Tools for Metabolic Syndrome among Apparently Healthy Ghanaian Adults." *Journal of Obesity* 2019 (September): 1–10. https://doi.org/10.1155/2019/8143179.

[104] Milagres, Luana Cupertino, Karina Oliveira Martinho, Diana Cupertino Milagres, Fernanda Silva Franco, Andréia Queiroz Ribeiro, and Juliana Farias de Novaes. 2019. "Relação Cintura/Estatura e Índice de Conicidade Estão Associados a Fatores de Risco Cardiometabólico Em Idosos." *Ciência & Saúde Coletiva* 24 (4): 1451–61. https://doi.org/10.1590/1413-81232018244.1263 2017. ["Waist / Height Ratio and Conicity Index Are Associated with Cardiometabolic Risk Factors In Elderly People." *Science & Collective Health*]

In: Anthropometry
Editor: Sébastien Legrand
ISBN: 978-1-53619-269-8
© 2021 Nova Science Publishers, Inc.

Chapter 2

ANTHROPOMETRY OF CHILDREN AGE 0-12 YEARS, IN THE SENEGAL RIVER VALLEY IN 1957: SITUATION AND PERSPECTIVES

Michel Garenne[1,2,3,4,*] *and Pierre Cantrelle*[5,†]

[1]Institut de Recherche pour le Développement (IRD),
UMI Résiliences, Bondy, France
[2]FERDI, Université d'Auvergne, Clermont-Ferrand, France
[3]Institut Pasteur, Épidémiologie des Maladies Émergentes,
Paris, France
[4]MRC/Wits Rural Public Health and Health Transitions Research Unit,
School of Public Health, Faculty of Health Sciences,
University of the Witwatersrand, Johannesburg
[5]Institut de Recherche pour le Développement (IRD),
Montpellier, France

---

[*] Corresponding Author's E-mail: mgarenne@hotmail.com.
[†] Corresponding Author's E-mail: pierrecantrelle@wanadoo.fr.

ABSTRACT

The anthropometry of children aged 0-12 years was studied during the multiple objectives survey conducted in the Middle Senegal River Valley (MISOES) in 1957-1958. This survey was based on two representative samples, in urban areas (769 children) and in rural areas (1240 children). Several measurements were taken: weight, height, arm circumference, triceps skinfold, subscapular skinfold, sub-iliac crest height, biacromial breadth, biiliac breadth. They were compared with American standards. Data show an overwhelming anthropometric deficit compared with standards, and complex interactions with age, gender, and place of residence. The average deficit, expressed as the percentage of reference values were: 80.6% for weight, 95.5% for height, 91.7% for body mass index (BMI), 78.6% for body surface area; it was more marked for triceps skinfold (67.6%) and for subscapular skinfold (66.3%), but less for arm circumference (84.9%) and for muscle circumference (87.7%); it was also marked for biacromial breadth (90.5%) and for biiliac breadth (91.9%), although keeping approximately constant the acromial-iliac ratio. Overall, deficits were more marked among children 1-2 years old, as well as among the 9-12 years old. Gender differences were not pronounced, but boys were somewhat disadvantaged before age 3 years, while girls were in greater deficit at age 9-12 years. Differences by place of residence were small and complex: deficits were higher in rural areas for skinfolds, but higher in urban areas for arm- and muscle- circumference. Results from the MISOES survey were put into perspective by comparing them with other studies also conducted in Senegal among under-five children: Niakhar (1983-1984) and DHS surveys (1993-2017). The relationships with economic development in the valley are discussed.

Keywords: anthropometry, children, weight, height, BMI, body surface, arm circumference, triceps skinfold, subscapular skinfold, biacromial breadth, biiliac breadth, iliac crest height, acromio-iliac index, MISOES, Niakhar, DHS surveys, Senegal, Senegal River valley

INTRODUCTION

The MISOES survey (Socio-economic Mission of the Senegal River Valley), was conducted in 1957-1958 along the Senegal river. This area is located in northern Senegal (left bank) and southern Mauritania (right bank). The survey was designed to inform future economic and social development programs in the years following independence (1960). It was a multi-purpose survey aiming at identifying demographic, health, economic and social problems in order to inform development policies and programs. These large-scale statistical surveys were pioneers at a time when there was little quantitative data on African populations, their demographic dynamics, their health profiles, and their levels of economic development. These surveys were initiated by the cooperation department of INSEE (the French National Institute of Statistics and Economic Studies). The MISOES survey was one of the first of these surveys, shortly following a similar survey in Côte d'Ivoire. They were followed by fifteen demographic surveys conducted in the former French-speaking African colonies in the 1960's and early 1970's. These demographic surveys were analyzed in summary documents (Groupe de Démographie Africaine, 1973a, 1973b, 1977).

The MISOES survey was conducted in the middle valley of the Senegal river, between Dembakane (upstream) and Dagana (downstream), on both banks of the river, over a length of about 400 km. It covered an estimated population of 341,000 inhabitants. It is described in detail in a reference book (Boutillier, Cantrelle et al. 1962). The study included several components: demography, health profile, household income, housing, land tenure, agriculture and food intake. The health component included morbidity, including local tropical diseases and disabilities, clinical and biological exams, as well as child anthropometry.

The anthropometric component of the survey was not analyzed in the documents published at the time. These data were archived by Pierre Cantrelle, in the form of detailed statistical tables, and are analyzed in this document. The anthropometric survey focused on children 0-12 years of both sexes. It was stratified into two groups (urban and rural), and focused on several parameters of child growth (weight, height), skeleton development (shoulders, hips, legs), as well as fat mass and muscle mass (arm circumference, triceps skinfold, subscapular skinfold).

1. DATA AND METHODS

1.1. Sample Size

The anthropometric survey covered about 10% of households in urban areas, and about 1.5% of households in rural areas. Comparing the age distribution of the anthropometric survey with that of the expected population shows that the age groups 0-8 years are well covered, but that the 9-12 years old are less well represented. However, the age patterns of the main nutritional parameters appeared regular, so that all ages from 0 to 12 years were considered in this analysis. In total, the sample included 769 children in urban areas and 1240 children in rural areas, numbers which allow numerous analyzes by sex, age and place of residence (Table 1).

Table 1. Sample size of the anthropometric survey, MISOES, 1957

Age (years)	Number surveyed (both sexes)		Number of children in the population		Sampling fraction (percent)	
	Urban	Rural	Urban	Rural	Urban	Rural
0-2	252	341	2684	29037	9.39%	1.17%
3-5	225	399	2149	23260	10.47%	1.72%
6-8	223	344	1910	20665	11.68%	1.66%
9-12	69	156	2299	24888	3.00%	0.63%
Total	769	1240	9042	97850	8.50%	1.27%

1.2. Anthropometric Measurements and Reference Standards

The anthropometric survey was comprehensive. It included several measures of child growth: weight and height; measurements of fat mass and muscle mass: arm circumference, triceps skinfold, subscapular skinfold; as well as skeletal growth measurements: shoulder width (biacromial breadth), hips width (iliac bi-crest breadth), and leg height (iliac sub-crest height). All the measures were taken by a well-trained operator (Mr. Mamadou Téra), from IFAN (French Institute for Black

Africa, Dakar), trained by Dr. Pierre Cantrelle (physician, anthropologist and nutritionist from IFAN), and integrated into the MISOES medical team under the supervision of a physician and nutritionist (Dr. Thianar N'doye) from ORANA (Office for Research on Food and Nutrition in Africa, Dakar).

The mean values of anthropometric measures by age observed in the MISOES survey were compared with reference values. It should be noted that the age data relate to the year of age (and not the age at birthday), so that the 'less than a year' category represents the age group '0-11 months', '1 year' the '12 -23 months' group, ..., and '12 years' the '132-143 months' group. As the differences between the sexes and between urban and rural areas were small, values of the deficits will be first presented for the whole population, focusing on the age patterns, then sex and urban/rural differences will be presented and discussed. For weight and height, the reference values were American standards, those of the CDC-2000, which are standards giving the median and standard deviation of weight by age, height by age and the body mass index (BMI) (CDC 2000). These standards were established from the NHANES anthropometric surveys, on representative samples of American children (NCHS, 1996). Since only values by year of age were available in the MISOES survey statistical tables, they were compared with the average by year of age of the CDC-2000 standards.

For arm circumference, triceps skinfold and subscapular skinfold, the standards were also American reference values, but taken directly from the NHANES-III survey, conducted in 1998-2004. These data provide the mean and standard deviation of these parameters by year of age. For the biacromial and biiliac breadths and the corresponding stature, the reference values were also taken from the NHANES-III survey, tabulated by sex and year of age. However, the NHANES-III survey did not provide the iliac crest height, but only the sitting height. The iliac crest height for the reference value was approximated by taking the difference between standing height and sitting height and adding 10% of the standing height (hip height). Comparisons with reference values were done for each sex separately. The average for boys and girls was taken for both sexes combined.

Several indicators were calculated from anthropometric measurements to assess the nutritional status of children in the MISOES survey, according to conventional formulas:

BMI = Weight/Height²

Where weight is in kg, height in m, and body mass index (BMI) in kg/m².

BSA = a × Weight^b × Taille^c

With a = 0.0235; b = 0.51456; c = 0.42246; where weight is in kg, height in cm and body surface area (BSA) in m².
Muscle circumference = Arm circumference − π × Triceps skinfold
Biacromial ratio = Biacromial breadth/Stature
Biiliac ratio = Biiliac breadth/Stature
Iliac sub-crest ratio = Iliac sub-crest height/Stature
Biacromial/biiliac index = Biacromial breadth/Biiliac breadth

2. RESULTS

2.1. Weight and Height

This section discusses weight, height and their combinations: weight/height ratio (body mass index) and body surface area. The formulas used for the calculations are presented in the methodological section.

2.1.1. Weight

Children's weights followed a fairly regular, almost linear, age pattern, ranging from 6.4 kg in children under one year of age, 18.1 kg in 6 years old children, to 30.0 kg in 12 years old children. The average weight was well below the reference standards, the average difference being 5.5 kg.

The difference was small in the first year of life (0.9 kg), then increased with age, widened beyond 9 years, reaching a maximum of 14.7 kg at 12 years of age. Expressed as a percentage of standards, the deficit appeared moderate in the first year of life (88.3%), then increased rapidly at 1-2 years (76.1%), before recovering and settling at a minimum at 7-8 years (86.1%), having almost recovered the initial level, before plunging again to reach its highest level at 11-12 years (71.7%). Two periods are therefore strongly weight-deficient: very young children (1-2 years) and pre-adolescents (10-12 years). All these deficits were highly statistically significant (Figure 1, Table 2).

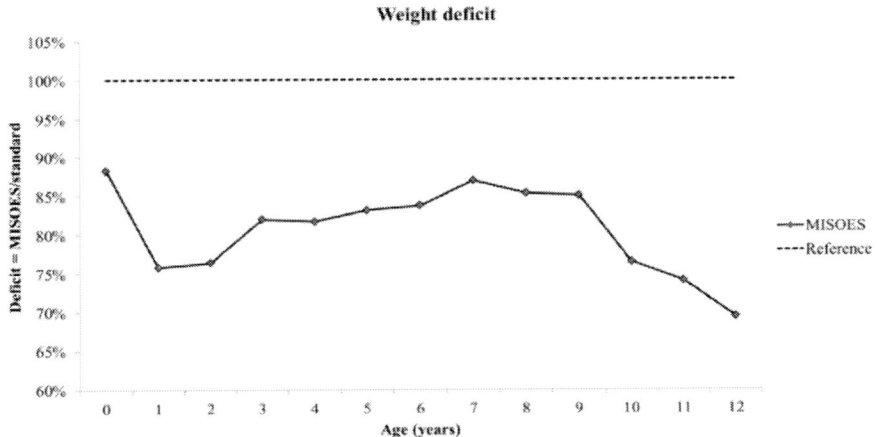

Figure 1. Weight deficit compared to standards, by age, MISOES, 1957.

The deficits were similar for both sexes before 9 years, and only the deficit of girls aged 9-12 was significantly greater than that of boys of the same age ($P = 0.032$). The weight deficit was also similar in urban and rural areas. The differences between urban and rural were not significant between 1 and 10 years, the deficit was greater in rural areas before 1 year ($P = 0.028$), and greater in urban areas at 11-12 years ($P = 0.016$), but these differences remained small (Table 2).

Table 2. Differentials in weight deficit compared to standards, MISOES, 1957

Category	Age group						
	< 1 year	1-2 years	3-4 years	5-6 years	7-8 years	9-10 years	11-12 years
Mean deficit							
Value	0.883	0.761	0.818	0.834	0.861	0.808	0.717
CI-min	0.853	0.748	0.805	0.823	0.847	0.787	0.696
CI-max	0.914*	0.775*	0.833*	0.846*	0.876*	0.829*	0.739*
By gender							
Boys	0.892	0.758	0.817	0.831	0.859	0.835	0.726
Girls	0.874	0.764	0.819	0.838	0.863	0.780	0.708
P-(diff)	0.571(ns)	0.701(ns)	0.889(ns)	0.510(ns)	0.821(ns)	0.010*	0.427(ns)
By area of residence							
Urban	0.922	0.771	0.831	0.843	0.866	0.808	0.681
Rural	0.853	0.756	0.812	0.831	0.859	0.799	0.734
P-(diff)	0.028*	0.284(ns)	0.167(ns)	0.312(ns)	0.666(ns)	0.687(ns)	0.016*

NB: Deficit = observed value/standard; P = value of the test of the difference between category; (ns) = not significant; (*) if P <0.05; CI-min/max = minimum and maximum value of the 95% confidence interval.

2.1.2. Height

Height also changed fairly regularly with age, ranging from 65.1 cm in children under 1 year old, to 114.3 cm in 6-year-olds, and 140.6 cm in 12-year-olds. Before 1 year, height was practically equal to that of the standard, then the gap widens, to recover a good part of the deficit at 7 years, before widening again until 12 years. Expressed as a percentage of the median of the reference values, the height of children under one year of age was comparable to standards, then stunting became strong at 1-4 years (93.6%), before recovering a good part at 7-8 years (97.3%), then plunging again to reach a strong deficit at 11-12 years (93.2%). Height changes were therefore similar to those of weight (Figure 2, Table 3).

Before 8 years of age the deficit was greater in boys, but the difference was significant only at 7-8 years of age (P = 0.019). The deficit reversed after 8 years, but differences between girls and boys remained small and not significant. The deficits were also similar in the two areas of residence, and no difference was significant before 11 years of age. The only significant difference was the greater deficit in urban areas at 11-12 years (P = 0.003), as for weight (Table 3).

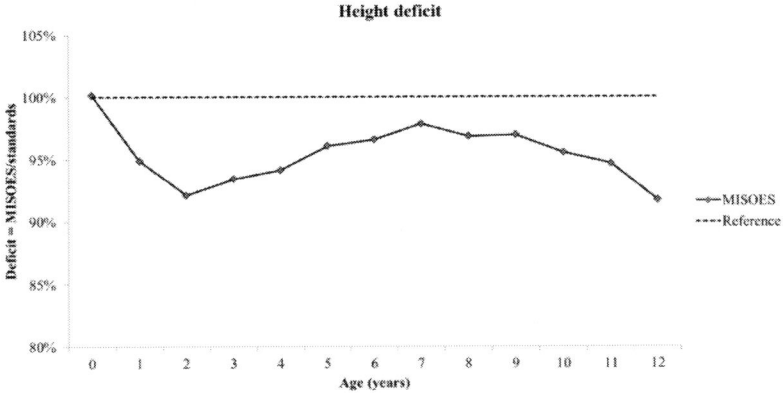

Figure 2. Height deficit compared to standards, by age, MISOES, 1957.

Table 3. Differentials in height deficit compared to standards, MISOES, 1957

Category	Age group						
	< 1 year	1-2 years	3-4 years	5-6 years	7-8 years	9-10 years	11-12 years
Mean deficit							
Value	1.001	0.935	0.938	0.963	0.973	0.962	0.932
CI-min	0.986	0.928	0.931	0.957	0.967	0.954	0.923
CI-max	1.016(ns)	0.942*	0.945*	0.969*	0.980*	0.971*	0.941*
By gender							
Boys	1.000	0.933	0.934	0.960	0.966	0.967	0.935
Girls	1.003	0.937	0.942	0.967	0.981	0.958	0.929
P-(diff)	0.851(ns)	0.638(ns)	0.319(ns)	0.263(ns)	0.019*	0.281(ns)	0.541(ns)
By area of residence							
Urban	1.010	0.938	0.946	0.965	0.974	0.954	0.908
Rural	0.994	0.934	0.934	0.963	0.973	0.963	0.942
P-(diff)	0.329(ns)	0.521(ns)	0.085(ns)	0.746(ns)	0.857(ns)	0.333(ns)	0.000*

NB: Deficit = observed value/standard; P = value of the test of the difference between category; (ns) = not significant; (*) if P <0.05; CI-min/max = minimum and maximum value of the 95% confidence interval.

2.1.3. The Weight/Height Ratio (BMI)

The body mass index (BMI), also known as the Quetelet index, measures relative leanness given size. The BMI of children in the MISOES survey did not follow the age pattern of the standards. Instead of increasing after 1 year, it decreased, then it decreased more sharply than expected, and finally it stagnated after age 9 years instead of increasing as expected from the standards. Compared with the standards, the deficit was already marked before 1 year (88.1%), then it decreased somewhat at 1-2 years (87.1%), before recovering in part at 3-4 years (93.0%), then it dropped slightly at 7-8 years (90.9%), then faster to reach its lowest values at 11-12 years (82.5%). The survey children were therefore always leaner than expected at equal height, especially at 0-1 years and 10-12 years. These two age groups combine both stunting and wasting (Figure 3).

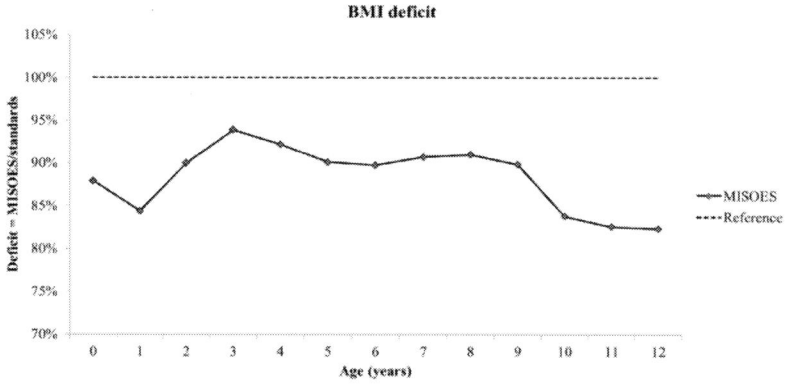

Figure 3. BMI deficit compared to standards, by age, MISOES, 1957.

The deficits in BMI were of the same order of magnitude for boys and girls, and if girls were always below boys, none of the differences was statistically significant. The same was true for the two areas of residence: changes in BMI were similar in both urban and rural areas, and no difference was statistically significant (Table 4).

Table 4. Differentials in deficit of the body mass index (BMI) compared to standards, MISOES, 1957

Category	Age group						
	< 1 year	1-2 years	3-4 years	5-6 years	7-8 years	9-10 years	11-12 years
Mean deficit							
Value	0.881	0.871	0.930	0.899	0.909	0.871	0.825
CI-min	0.841	0.852	0.909	0.882	0.890	0.844	0.796
CI-max	0.923*	0.891*	0.952*	0.916*	0.928*	0.899*	0.855*
By gender							
Boys	0.892	0.871	0.937	0.902	0.921	0.892	0.831
Girls	0.870	0.871	0.924	0.897	0.897	0.850	0.819
P-(diff)	0.297(ns)	0.954(ns)	0.284(ns)	0.461(ns)	0.134(ns)	0.614(ns)	0.060(ns)
By area of residence							
Urban	0.904	0.877	0.929	0.905	0.912	0.887	0.826
Rural	0.863	0.869	0.931	0.896	0.907	0.861	0.828
P-(diff)	0.323(ns)	0.678(ns)	0.930(ns)	0.603(ns)	0.809(ns)	0.397(ns)	0.968(ns)

NB: Deficit = observed value/standard; P = value of the test of the difference between category; (ns) = not significant; (*) if P <0.05; CI-min/max = minimum and maximum value of the 95% confidence interval.

2.1.4. Body Surface Area

The measurement of body surface area, on the contrary, presents a synthesis of child growth, since it combines both weight and height. Its age pattern therefore follows the combination of the two components. This age pattern was regular: it started from a value close to standards before 1 year (0.36 m²), to reach 0.77 m² at 6 years, and 1.09 m² at 12 years. Expressed as a percentage of standards, the deficit appeared small before 1 year (93.8%), then widened rapidly at 1-2 years (84.5%), to recover quickly reaching 91.6% at 7-8 years, before widening again and reaching its maximum at 11-12 years (81.8%). The weight and height deficit was therefore high in this population, especially at 1-2 years and at 11-12 years (Figure 4, Table 5).

The deficit was practically the same for boys and girls up to 7-8 years of age, however it was higher for girls between 9 and 12 years of age (P = 0.021). The differences between the two areas of residence were not significant between 1 and 10 years; the deficit was more marked in rural before 1 year (P = 0.016) and more marked in urban at 11-12 years (P = 0.001) (Table 5).

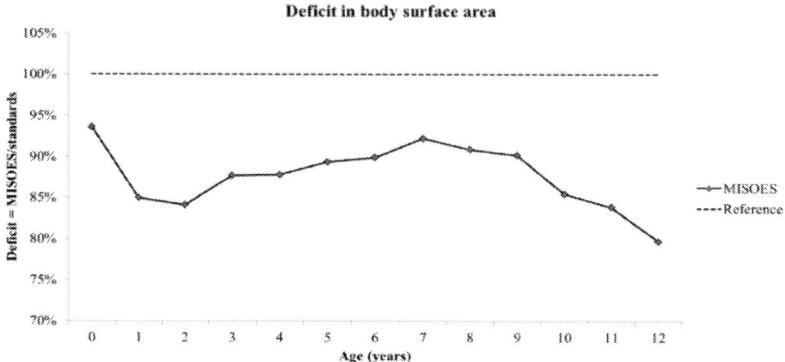

Figure 4. Deficit of body surface area compared to standards, by age, MISOES, 1957.

Table 5. Differentials in deficit in body surface area (BMI) compared to standards, MISOES, 1957

Category	Age group						
	< 1 year	1-2 years	3-4 years	5-6 years	7-8 years	9-10 years	11-12 years
Mean deficit							
Value	0.938	0.845	0.878	0.897	0.916	0.881	0.818
CI-min	0.921	0.837	0.870	0.890	0.907	0.869	0.805
CI-max	0.956*	0.853*	0.886*	0.904*	0.924*	0.893*	0.831*
By gender							
Boys	0.943	0.842	0.876	0.893	0.912	0.898	0.824
Girls	0.934	0.847	0.880	0.900	0.919	0.864	0.812
P-(diff)	0.640(ns)	0.611(ns)	0.633(ns)	0.311(ns)	0.379(ns)	0.006*	0.353(ns)
By area of residence							
Urban	0.963	0.851	0.888	0.902	0.918	0.879	0.788
Rural	0.919	0.841	0.873	0.895	0.914	0.877	0.832
P-(diff)	0.016*	0.221(ns)	0.060(ns)	0.289(ns)	0.643(ns)	0.908(ns)	0.001*

NB: Deficit = observed value/standard; P = value of the test of the difference between category; (ns) = not significant; (*) if P <0.05; CI-min/max = minimum and maximum value of the 95% confidence interval.

2.1.5. Summary on Weight and Height Deficits

Figure 5 summarizes the weight and height deficits of children in the MISOES survey. All ages combined, the height deficit amounted to 95.5% of standards, the weight by height deficit to 91.7%, which produced almost equivalent deficits in weight by age (80.6%) and in body surface area (78.6%).

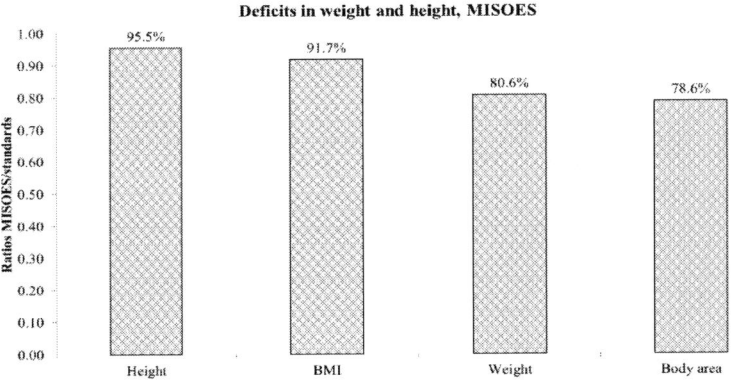

Figure 5. Synthesis of deficits in weight and height, children age 0-12 years, MISOES, 1957.

3.1. Fat Mass and Muscle Mass

This section presents the deficits in arm- and muscle- circumference, and in triceps- and subscapular- skinfolds, in order to estimate fat and muscle mass.

3.1.1. Arm Circumference

The average arm circumference in the MISOES sample was well below standards from the first years of life, and even more after 10 years. The development was not regular, and was similar for boys and girls, as well as for both areas of residence. The average deficit of arm circumference compared to the reference values was 89.3% before 1 year, then decreased to reach 83.3% at 7-8 years, then plunged and reached 78.8% at 11-12 years. (Figure 6, Table 6).

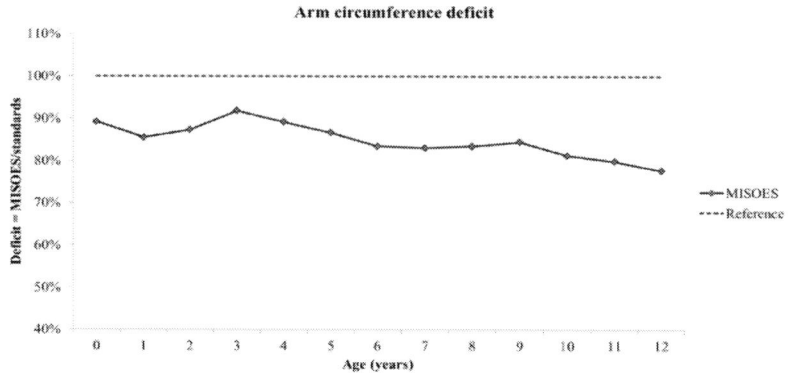

Figure 6. Arm circumference deficit compared to standards, by age, MISOES, 1957.

Table 6. Differentials in arm circumference deficit compared to standards, MISOES, 1957

Category	Age group						
	< 1 year	1-2 years	3-4 years	5-6 years	7-8 years	9-10 years	11-12 years
Mean deficit							
Value	0.893	0.865	0.905	0.851	0.833	0.830	0.788
CI-min	0.868	0.850	0.895	0.844	0.825	0.818	0.772
CI-max	0.918*	0.880*	0.916*	0.858*	0.842*	0.842*	0.805*
By gender							
Boys	0.903	0.862	0.891	0.839	0.819	0.824	0.787
Girls	0.882	0.867	0.920	0.862	0.848	0.835	0.789
P-(diff)	0.401(ns)	0.748(ns)	0.006*	0.001*	0.001*	0.366(ns)	0.907(ns)
By area of residence							
Urban	0.877	0.856	0.896	0.842	0.810	0.824	0.748
Rural	0.907	0.873	0.911	0.857	0.841	0.832	0.804
P-(diff)	0.229(ns)	0.241(ns)	0.139(ns)	0.041*	0.000*	0.541(ns)	0.002*

NB: Deficit = observed value/standard; P = value of the test of the difference between category; (ns) = not significant; (*) if P <0.05; CI-min/max = minimum and maximum value of the 95% confidence interval.

Girls had an advantage over boys between 1 and 10 years, significantly between 3 and 8 years, but the differences between the two sexes remained small, at 1.4% on average. The arm circumference deficit was more marked in urban areas (83.3%) than in rural areas (85.7%), with no interaction with age. These differences were significant in certain age groups (5-8 years, 11-12 years) but disappeared in others (0-4 years, to 9-

10 years). Overall, these differences between urban and rural were small, 2.4% on average (Table 6).

3.1.2. Triceps Skinfold

The average triceps skinfold followed a regular, but unexpected, change with age, and was much below standards at all ages. There were several anomalies: it was abnormally weak at 1-2 years, and it did not re-increase with age beyond 8 years, as would be expected by standards. The triceps skinfold deficit was fairly stable between 0 and 4 years, varying from 85.6% to 88.2%, then it increased with age from 5 years, reaching a very high value at 11-12 years (46.6%). Therefore, pre-adolescents (7-12 years) had a particularly low fat mass (Figure 7).

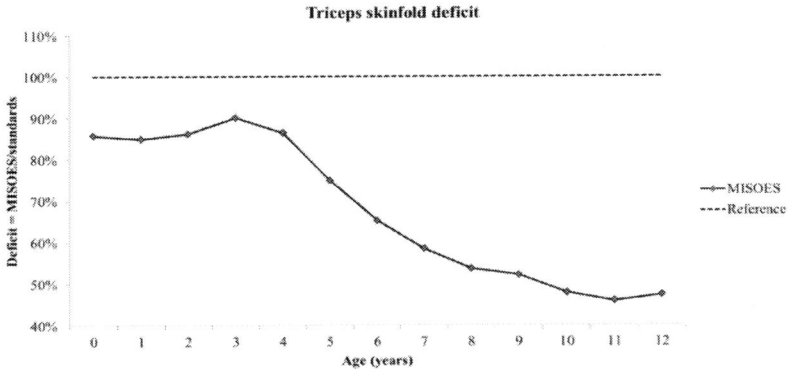

Figure 7. Triceps skinfold deficit compared to standards, by age, MISOES, 1957.

The deficit was practically the same for girls and boys before 8 years, and slightly higher for girls at 9-12 years, the difference being significant (P = 0.036). The age pattern of the deficit was similar in the two areas of residence. The rural environment was somewhat disadvantaged at all ages, with a greater deficit in the triceps skinfold (66.2%) than the urban environment (70.4%). The difference between urban and rural areas was noticeable before 1 year (P = 0.001), small and not significant between 1 and 4 years, greater thereafter and maximum at 9-12 years (P <0.001) (Table 7).

Table 7. Differentials of the triceps skinfold deficit compared to standards, MISOES, 1957

Category	Age group						
	< 1 year	1-2 years	3-4 years	5-6 years	7-8 years	9-10 years	11-12 years
Mean deficit							
Value	0.857	0.856	0.882	0.701	0.561	0.500	0.466
CI-min	0.833	0.840	0.865	0.685	0.546	0.478	0.441
CI-max	0.883*	0.872*	0.900*	0.716*	0.575*	0.523*	0.493*
By gender							
Boys	0.861	0.845	0.886	0.709	0.553	0.476	0.457
Girls	0.854	0.867	0.879	0.692	0.568	0.524	0.475
P-(diff)	0.786(ns)	0.177(ns)	0.705(ns)	0.273(ns)	0.277(ns)	0.023*	0.432(ns)
By area of residence							
Urban	0.907	0.864	0.888	0.718	0.588	0.580	0.484
Rural	0.820	0.849	0.882	0.686	0.548	0.473	0.458
P-(diff)	0.001*	0.368(ns)	0.752(ns)	0.043*	0.006*	0.000*	0.358(ns)

NB: Deficit = observed value/standard; P = value of the test of the difference between category; (ns) = not significant; (*) if P <0.05; CI-min/max = minimum and maximum value of the 95% confidence interval.

3.1.3. Subscapular Skinfold

The subscapular skinfold also followed a regular, but unexpected, pattern by age, as for the triceps skinfold. It remained fairly close to standards up to 4 years, then the gap from the reference values widened, the average skinfold remaining approximately constant afterwards, with little difference between sexes or between areas of residence, whereas it was expected to increase rapidly, especially in girls. The average deficit of the subscapular skinfold was moderate before 1 year (91.7%), then it decreased moderately to reach 81.0% at 3-4 years, before plunging rapidly to reach 45.3% at 11-12 years (Figure 8; Table 8).

The deficits were similar in girls and in boys between 3 and 12 years, but higher in girls before 1 year (P <0.001) and at 1-4 years (P = 0.023). The average deficit of the subscapular skinfold was always greater in rural areas than in urban areas, and changes with age were approximately parallel, the average difference being +4.3%, the differences being significant in each age group 0-10, but not at 11-12 years (Table 8).

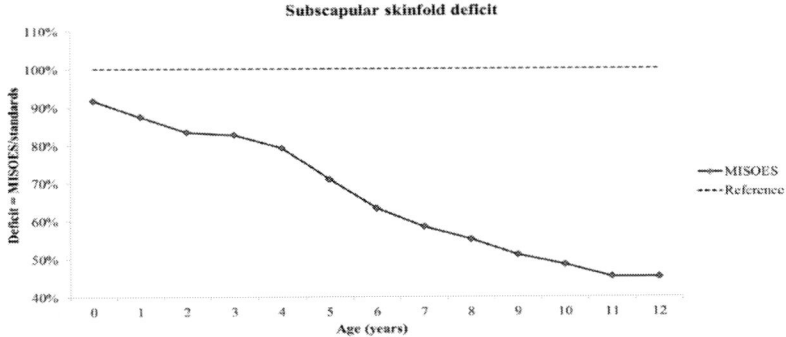

Figure 8. Subscapular skinfold deficit compared to standards, by age, MISOES, 1957.

Table 8. Differentials of the sub-scapular skinfold deficit compared to standards, MISOES, 1957

Category	Age group						
	< 1 year	1-2 years	3-4 years	5-6 years	7-8 years	9-10 years	11-12 years
Mean deficit							
Value	0.917	0.854	0.810	0.671	0.568	0.498	0.453
CI-min	0.884	0.838	0.793	0.658	0.557	0.478	0.433
CI-max	0.951*	0.871*	0.828*	0.684*	0.580*	0.518*	0.473*
By gender							
Boys	0.999	0.873	0.815	0.680	0.577	0.497	0.471
Girls	0.834	0.836	0.806	0.663	0.560	0.498	0.434
P-(diff)	0.000*	0.023*	0.628(ns)	0.201(ns)	0.126(ns)	0.972(ns)	0.054(ns)
By area of residence							
Urban	0.959	0.875	0.838	0.693	0.591	0.541	0.467
Rural	0.876	0.831	0.796	0.654	0.557	0.481	0.446
P-(diff)	0.017*	0.007*	0.019*	0.005*	0.004*	0.011*	0.377(ns)

NB: Deficit = observed value/standard; P = value of the test of the difference between category; (ns) = not significant; (*) if P <0.05; CI-min/max = minimum and maximum value of the 95% confidence interval.

3.1.4. Muscle Circumference

Muscle circumference results from the difference between arm circumference and triceps skinfold. Therefore, muscle circumference followed a pattern similar to arm circumference, but with a smaller difference from standards due to the impact of the skinfold. The evolution by age was fairly regular: a slight increase between 0 and 1 year, some recovery afterwards, with little difference between sexes and between places of residence. Expressed as a percentage of the reference values, the deficit appeared fairly constant according to age, with small fluctuations, going from 90.2% before 1 year, 86.7% at 1-2 years, 91.0% at 3-4 years and 85.9% at 11-12 years (Figure 9, Table 9).

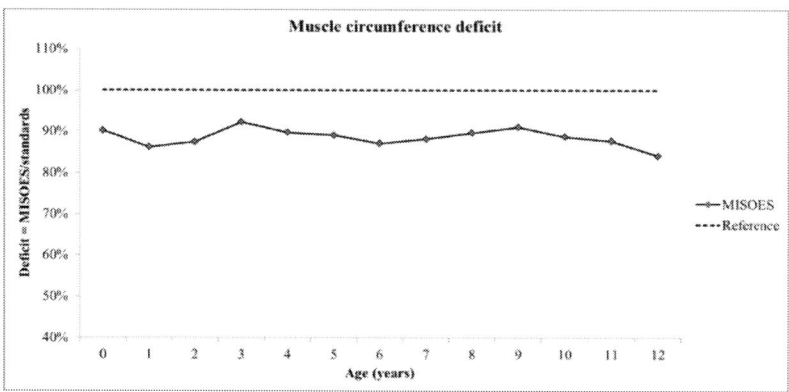

Figure 9. Deficit of muscle circumference compared to standards, by age, MISOES, 1957.

Table 9. Differentials in muscle circumference compared to standards, MISOES, 1957

Category	Age group						
	< 1 year	1-2 years	3-4 years	5-6 years	7-8 years	9-10 years	11-12 years
Mean deficit							
Value	0.902	0.867	0.910	0.881	0.889	0.901	0.859
CI-min	0.893	0.862	0.906	0.878	0.886	0.895	0.853
CI-max	0.911*	0.871*	0.915*	0.885*	0.893*	0.906*	0.866*
By gender							
Boys	0.915	0.866	0.892	0.864	0.869	0.893	0.854
Girls	0.890	0.867	0.929	0.899	0.910	0.908	0.865
P-(diff)	0.005*	0.860(ns)	0.000*	0.000*	0.000*	0.002*	0.073(ns)
By area of residence							
Urban	0.869	0.854	0.898	0.867	0.856	0.877	0.806
Rural	0.930	0.879	0.917	0.891	0.901	0.909	0.880
P-(diff)	0.000*	0.000*	0.000*	0.000*	0.000*	0.000*	0.000*

NB: Deficit = observed value/standard; P = value of the test of the difference between category; (ns) = not significant; (*) if P <0.05; CI-min/max = minimum and maximum value of the 95% confidence interval.

Differences by sex were small, 4.1% on average, the deficit being always more marked in boys, and differences being significant between 3 and 8 years. The muscle circumference deficit was more marked in urban than in rural, and significantly so at all ages, but remained of small magnitude: 5.1% on average (Table 9).

3.1.5. Summary on Subcutaneous Fat and Muscle Mass Deficits

In summary, the differentials of subcutaneous fat and muscle were notable. Deficits were strong for skinfolds (66.3% and 67.6%), but moderate for muscles (87.7%) (Figure 10).

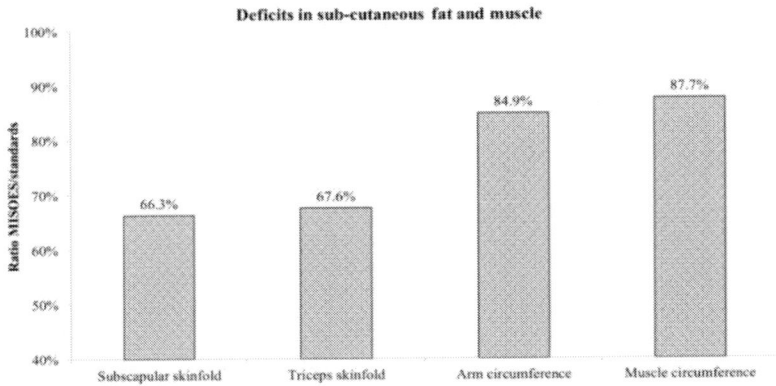

Figure 10. Summary on skinfold and muscle deficits, children 0-12 years old, MISOES.

4.1. Body Morphology

This section presents three measures of skeletal development: the length of the legs (iliac crest height), the shoulder width (biacromial breadth) and the hips width (iliac bi-crest width), presented in relation to the stature.

4.1.1. Iliac Crest Height (Legs)

The iliac crest height followed a fairly regular evolution by age, with little difference between girls and boys, nor between urban and rural areas.

The average length of legs was practically identical to that of reference American children at all ages, while the stature was much lower, which shows a different body shape for Sahelian children, as indeed for adults (longer legs in relation to the body). The ratio of iliac crest height to stature was therefore always higher than that of American children. In addition, it was not constant with age: it decreased between 2 and 5 years, which shows a delay in the development of the upper part of the body, then it evolved normally thereafter, slightly increasing until 11-12 years. There were no differences in the ratio between boys and girls, nor between urban and rural areas (Figure 11, Table 10).

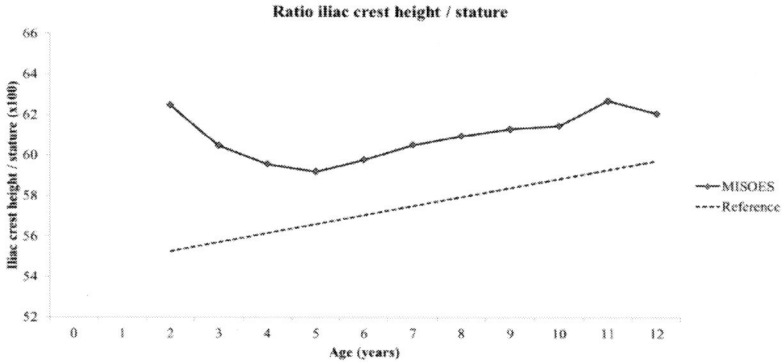

Figure 11. Ratio of iliac crest height/stature, by age, MISOES, 1957.

Table 10. Elements of morphology in relation to standards, MISOES, 1957

Category	Age group						
	< 1 year	1-2 years	3-4 years	5-6 years	7-8 years	9-10 years	11-12 years
Ratio iliac crest height/stature							
MISOES		62.48	59.99	59.49	60.71	61.47	62.37
Deficit/excess		1.13	1.07	1.05	1.05	1.05	1.05
Ratio biacromial breadth/stature							
MISOES	23.52	21.51	22.25	21.63	21.37	21.20	21.09
Deficit		0.94	0.98	0.96	0.96	0.96	0.96

Category	Age group						
	< 1 year	1-2 years	3-4 years	5-6 years	7-8 years	9-10 years	11-12 years
Ratio biiliac breadth/stature							
MISOES	16.42	15.47	16.28	15.56	15.13	14.89	14.86
Deficit		0.95	1.02	0.98	0.97	0.96	0.96
Acromio-iliac index							
MISOES	69.82	71.92	73.14	71.96	70.83	70.23	70.49
Deficit/excess		1.02	1.04	1.02	1.01	1.00	1.01

NB: Deficit/excess = Observed value/standard.

4.1.2. Biacromial Breadth (Shoulders)

The biacromial breadth of MISOES children was well below American standards. It evolved roughly parallel with age, but with a more marked deficit at 2 years and at 11-12 years, as was the case for stature. There were little differences by sex or by place of residence. The ratio of biacromial breadth to stature decreased with age, as in American standards. It was always lower in the MISOES data, indicating a slower development of shoulders compared with stature, and especially at 1-2 years, with a rapid recovery at 3-4 years (Figure 12, Table 10).

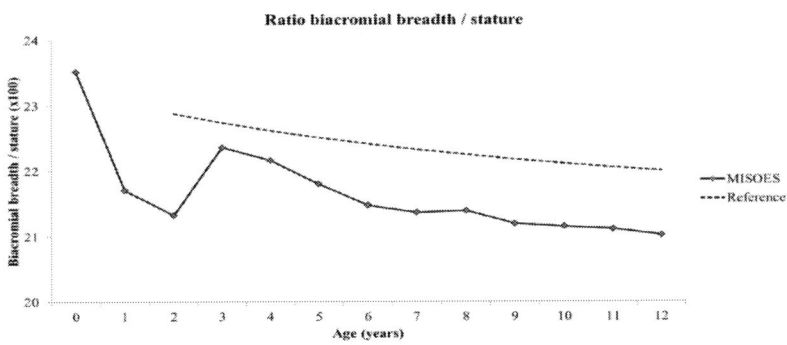

Figure 12. Ratio of biacromial breadth to stature, and comparison with standards, by age, MISOES, 1957.

4.1.3. Biiliac Breadth (Hips)

Biiliac breadth evolved similarly. The evolution by age was fairly regular, but with a larger gap from standards at 2 years, as well as at 11-12 years, with little difference by sex or by place of residence.

The ratio of biiliac breadth to stature decreased with age, as in the American reference. As for shoulders, the development of the hips in relation to stature was slower at 1-2 years, with a rapid recovery at 3-4 years, reaching even a value greater than the American reference for a few years (Figure 13, Table 10).

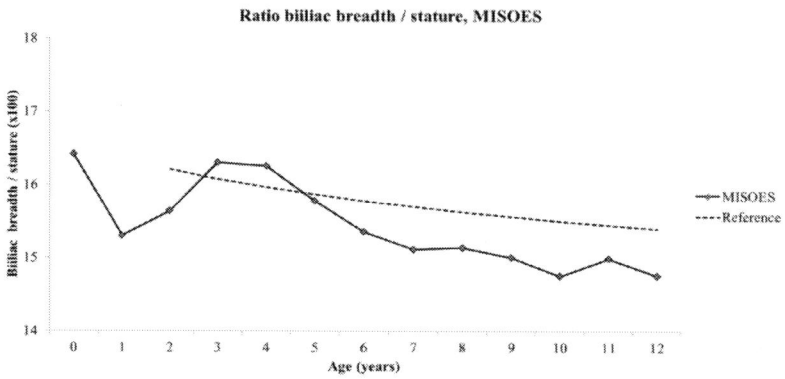

Figure 13. Ratio of biiliac breadth to stature and comparison with standards, by age, MISOES, 1957.

4.1.4. Acromio-Iliac Index

The acromio-iliac index measures the shoulders width relative to that of the hips. This index is fairly constant by age in American standards, with a slight decrease by age. Among children of the Senegal River valley, the relationship evolved differently: an increase of the ratio between 0 and 2 years, followed by a decrease thereafter, which indicates that the hips was disadvantaged at first compared to the shoulders, before stabilizing. Differences by sex were small before 9 years of age, but the gap widened between 9 and 12 years of age, with girls having a significantly higher index. As the two measures composing the index were below standards, this means that the enlargement of the girls' hips was less important than expected at 9-12 years (Figure 14, Table 10).

Anthropometry of Children Age 0-12 Years ... 61

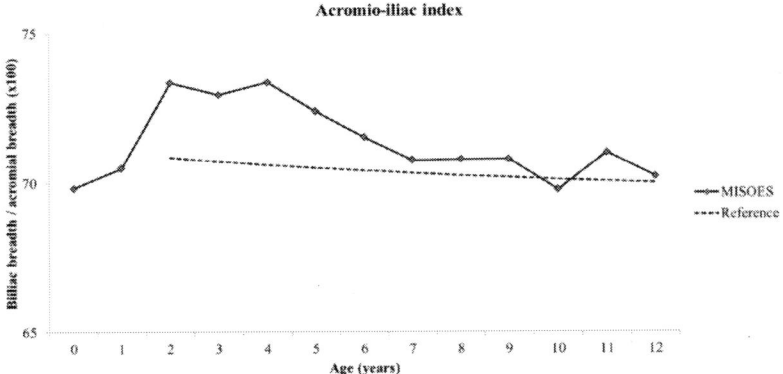

Figure 14. Acromio-iliac index and comparison with standards, by age, MISOES, 1957.

4.1.5. Synthesis on Body Morphology

Figure 15 presents the main skeletal deficits compared with American references: 95.5% in height, 91.9% in biiliac breadth and 90.5% in biacromial breadth, approximately respecting the acromio-iliac ratio. On the other hand, the leg length did not present a deficit.

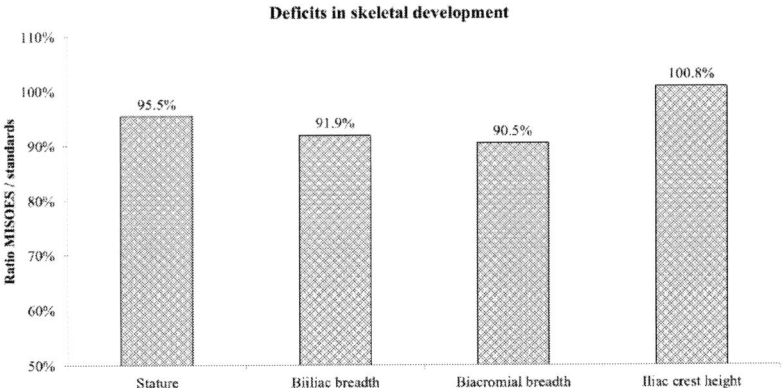

Figure 15. Summary on skeletal development deficits, children 2-12 years old, MISOES.

5.1. Summary: Differentials in Children's Anthropometry

5.1.1. Differences According to Anthropometric Indicators

The nutritional status of young children in the Senegal valley was therefore in net deficit, practically for all measures and at all ages, except the height of children under one year of age and the leg length at all ages. This was true for height-for-age, for weight-for-height (BMI), and therefore for weight-for-age and for body surface area; as for muscle circumference and the skinfolds, and therefore for arm circumference; as for the width of hips and shoulders relative to stature. The order of magnitude of the deficits varied according to the indicator chosen and to age. The most sensitive indicators were the skinfolds and weight-for-age, and the most stable were skeletal indicators. Two age groups were particularly prone to deficit: 1-4 years (and especially 1-2 years) and 9-12 years (and especially 11-12 years), as seen above and summarized in the following table (Table 11).

Table 11. Average anthropometric deficits in children 0-12 years old, MISOES, 1957

	Height	Weight for height = BMI	Muscle circum-ference	Skinfolds	Biacromial ratio	Biiliac ratio
Total	95.5%	91.7%	87.7%	67.0%	90.5%	91.9%
<1 year	100.1%	88.1%	90.2%	88.7%		
1-4 years	93.6%	90.1%	88.9%	85.1%	88.8%	91.8%
5-8 years	96.8%	90.4%	88.5%	62.5%	93.1%	94.4%
9-12 years	94.7%	84.7%	87.9%	47.9%	89.2%	89.5%

NB: Skinfolds = average of the triceps and subscapular skinfold.

5.1.2. Differences between Girls and Boys

Differences between girls and boys were generally small for most indicators. Few other indicators were available for comparison. The only other indicator available in the MISOES survey was the mortality of young children. The under-five mortality quotient, (under-five deaths/live births), was almost identical for boys and girls (322 versus 319 per 1,000), the difference being not significant. This observation could be linked to sex differences in arm-circumference of under-five children, the most sensitive anthropometric indicator for mortality: arm circumference compared with American standards was practically identical for girls and boys. However, several significant differences were noted above, and are summarized in the following table. Girls aged 9-12 appeared somewhat disadvantaged in weight and body surface area, but boys appeared somewhat disadvantaged in muscle (all ages), in triceps skinfold (9-12 years) and in arm circumference (5-8 years). In any case, there was no systematic difference that could have indicated any discrimination against one or the other sex (Table 12).

Table 12. Main significant differences in deficits between girls and boys, MISOES, 1957

Deficit indicator, age group	Boys	Girls	Difference (B-G)	P-value
Weight, 9-12 years	78.0%	74.4%	+3.6%	0.032*
Body surface area, 9-12 years	86.1%	83.8%	+2.3%	0.021*
Muscle circumference, all ages	85.7%	89.8%	−4.1%	0.000*
Triceps skinfold, 9-12 years	46.6%	50.0%	−3.3%	0.036*
Arm circumference, 5-8 years	82.9%	85.5%	−2.6%	0.000*

5.1.3. Differences between Urban and Rural Areas

Differences between the two areas of residence were more contrasted, although of small magnitude. On one hand, the urban environment appeared slightly disadvantaged in height and surface, as well as in arm- and muscle- circumference, but not in weight-for-height. On the other hand, the rural environment appeared disadvantaged in both, triceps- and subscapular- skinfolds (Table 13).

These differences could be linked to other indicators of the health status of urban and rural populations. The MISOES survey provides data on fertility, mortality and morbidity by place of residence (Table 14). Fertility, measured by complete family size among women aged 50-69 years, was slightly higher in rural areas. Mortality, measured by under-five mortality, was slightly higher in urban areas. Severe malnutrition, measured by the prevalence of kwashiorkor was much higher in rural areas, as well as the prevalence of malaria, measured by splenomegaly. However, the prevalence of clinical anemia was higher in urban areas. The urban environment was therefore penalized by anemia and infant and child mortality, which is consistent with the lower arm- and muscle-circumference, which were also lower in urban areas. Conversely, the higher prevalence of kwashiorkor in rural areas is consistent with the higher deficit in skinfolds in rural areas.

Table 13. Main significant differences between urban and rural areas, MISOES, 1957

Deficit indicator, age	Urban	Rural	Difference (U-R)	P-value
Height, 9-12 years	93.1%	95.3%	−2.2%	0.003*
Body surface area, 9-12 years	83.3%	85.4%	−2.1%	0.035*
Arm circumference, all ages	83.3%	85.7%	−2.4%	0.000*
Muscle circumference, all ages	84.5%	89.6%	−5.1%	0.000*
Triceps skinfold, all ages	70.4%	66.2%	+4.2%	0.000*
Subscapular skinfold, all ages	69.0%	64.7%	+4.3%	0.000*

Table 14. Differences between urban and rural areas for other indicators, MISOES, 1957

Health indicator	Urban	Rural	Difference (U−R)	P-value
Demographic indicator				
Retrospective fertility (children ever-born/woman)	4.95	5.20	−0.25	0.036*
Retrospective mortality (deaths 0-4 years/1000 births)	379	358	+22	0.001*
Prevalence per 100 children				
Malaria morbidity (splenomegaly)	4.7%	37.8%	−33.1%	<0.001*
Clinical anemia	34.2%	27.1%	+7.1%	ND
Kwashiorkor	0.5%	2.3%	−1.8%	ND

NB. Samples size for anemia and kwashiorkor were not available, so testing differences could not be done.

6.1. Comparison with the Anthropometry of Children Aged 0-4 Years in Niakhar (1983-1984)

The MISOES anthropometric data were compared with data collected by the same group from ORSTOM (now IRD) in Niakhar, a study area located in the groundnut basin in central Senegal (Fatick region), where a health and demographic surveillance system is in place since 1962 (Cantrelle 1969; Garenne & Cantrelle 1989, 1997; Garenne et al. 2018). The Niakhar area is located in a different ecological zone, the Sudano-Sahelian tree savannah. During the anthropometric study conducted in Niakhar in 1983-1984, the level of infant and child mortality (285 per 1000) was of the same order of magnitude, although a little lower, than that observed in the river valley in 1957-1958 (322 per 1000). Living conditions were somewhat different, the main differences being the presence of the river and the abundance of fish in the valley, as well as the possibility of irrigated cultivation, making the area less sensitive to climatic hazards. The Niakhar study included several comparable anthropometric measurements: weight, height, arm circumference, triceps- and subscapular- skinfolds, but no skeletal measurement, and was restricted to under-five children. The Niakhar study was carried out during the drought years (1983-1984), which were difficult years of food scarcity, but where food aid was abundant (Garenne et al. 2000).

Overall, the anthropometric measures taken in the river valley were rather lower than those in the Niakhar area, but not for all measures (Table 15, Figure 16). Considering the anthropometry of children 2-4 years old, deficits were more marked in the river valley in height (98.3%), body surface area (94.2%), BMI (93.4%), and weight (91.3%). Age patterns were fairly consistent, although before the age of 1 year, the differences between the two studies were small, as the two study areas were close to international standards at this age. This indicates that the profile of stunting and recovery was quite similar in the two cases, but that stunting and wasting were more pronounced in the Senegal River valley. This observation goes in the same direction as the difference in mortality, which was slightly higher in the valley.

Table 15. Ratio of MISOES measurements (1957-1958) to Niakhar measurements (1983-1984)

Measurement	Age (years)				
	< 1 year	1 an	2 years	3 years	4 years
Weight & Height					
Height-for-age	1.013	0.999	0.982	0.983	0.985
Weight-for-height (BMI)	0.944	0.959	0.931	0.933	0.937
Weight-for-age	0.969	0.957	0.897	0.901	0.909
Surface-area/age	0.989	0.977	0.938	0.941	0.946
Arm & skinfolds					
Muscle circumference	0.994	1.012	1.032	1.066	1.044
Arm circumference	1.012	1.013	1.011	1.038	1.032
Triceps skinfold	1.086	1.016	0.921	0.916	0.975
Subscapular skinfold	0.978	1.007	0.933	0.917	0.975

For the measurements of fat mass and muscle mass, the differences were more contrasted. Children in the Senegal River valley had similar measures before the age of 2 years. Beyond this age, the skinfolds were lower than those in the Niakhar area, especially at 2-3 years, which is consistent with differences in weight-for-age, but arm- and muscle-circumference were higher. Therefore, despite their deficit in fat mass, the valley children had more muscle. This could be due to differences in diet between the two areas.

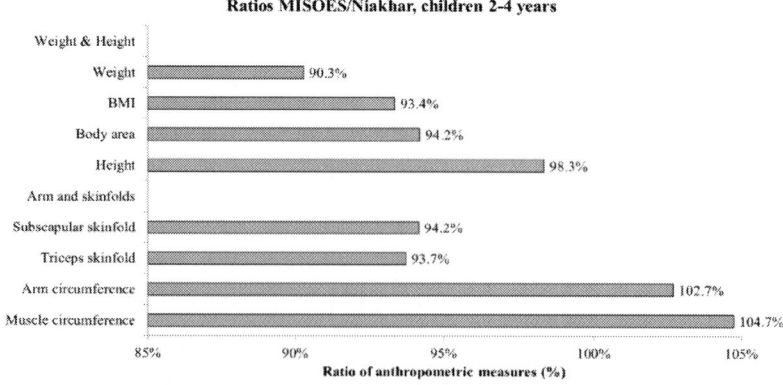

Figure 16. Ratio of anthropometric measurements MISOES/Niakhar, children 2-4 years old.

7.1. Future of the Population: Comparison with DHS Surveys (1993-2017)

The 1957 MISOES data were put into perspective by comparing them with the long-term trends provided by the Demographic and Health Surveys (DHS). Eight DHS surveys measured the anthropometry of children under five (weight and height), conducted in 1993, 2005, 2011, 2013, 2014, 2015, 2016, 2017. For the comparison, the same region was selected, the River valley area, currently including the Saint-Louis and Matam regions, and selecting rural areas. These surveys totaled 4803 children, including 977 four-year-olds.

DHS surveys showed an increase in height and weight of under-five children between 1993 and 2017. A linear regression over survey year, and controlling for age, gave significant coefficients, for height (b = +0.0949; P < 0.00001) and for weight (b = +0.0073; P = 0.025). The 4-year-olds were selected for further comparison, since they best summarize trends in weight and the height. For this age group, the trend was significant for height (b = +0.1814; P < 0.00001), but not for weight (b = +0.0144; P = 0.084), even though the coefficient remained positive. In summary, in 24 years between 1993 and 2017, children aged 48-59 months grew a lot, gaining 4.4 cm in height, but gained little weight, only 350 g.

The comparison of MISOES data with DHS data indicates that the height of 4-year-old children stagnated for a long time, even declining slightly between 1957 (98.7 cm) and 1993 (97.7 cm), before increasing rapidly thereafter, to reach 101.9 cm in 2014-2017, still remaining far from American standards (105.4 cm), but having made up about half of their deficit. Their weight remained stable for a long time at 14.2 kg, and increased only in the most recent period (14.5 kg), but remained far from American standards (18.1 kg). Consequently, their BMI initially increased slightly, from 14.1 kg/m² in 1957 to 14.8 kg/m² in 1993, before falling rapidly, to reach 14.0 kg/m² in 2014-2017, a strong deficit compared to American standards (16.3 kg/m²) (Figure 17, Table 16). This evolution in the river valley, with increasing height but decreasing BMI, is parallel to the evolution of these parameters throughout the country (Garenne 2018, 2020).

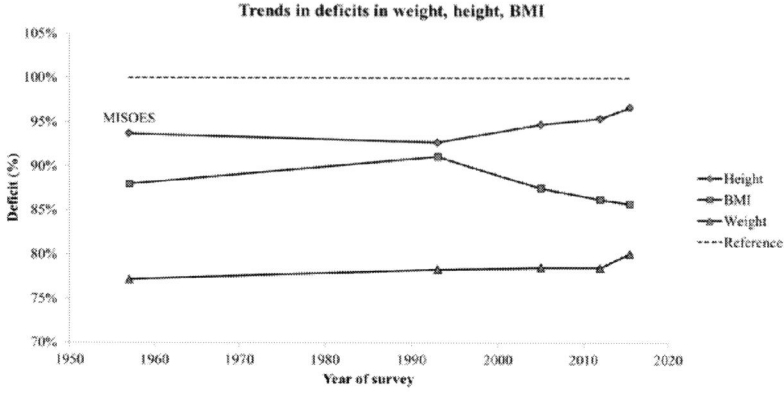

Figure 17. Trends in weight and height deficits, children age 4 years, Senegal River Valley, 1957-2017.

Table 16. Trends in anthropometry of 4-year-old children, Senegal River Valley, 1957-2017

Survey year	Mean values at 48-59 months			Deficits with respect to USA standards		
	Weight (kg)	Height (cm)	BMI (kg/m^2)	Weight	Height	BMI
1957	13.95	98.73	14.31	77.2%	93.7%	88.0%
1993	14.15	97.73	14.82	78.3%	92.7%	91.1%
2005	14.19	99.85	14.23	78.5%	94.7%	87.5%
2012	14.19	100.57	14.03	78.5%	95.4%	86.2%
2016	14.48	101.88	13.95	80.1%	96.7%	85.7%

NB: 1957 = MISOES; 1993-2017 = DHS surveys. The 2011-2013 surveys, and 2014-2017 surveys were grouped together.

8.1. Relationship with Economic Development

The evolution in the anthropometry of under-five children could be linked to economic and climatic changes in the region. In 1957, the Senegal River valley was a poor and remote area, living mainly from traditional agriculture (crops, livestock, fishing) and a little trade. The area was semi-arid and sensitive to climatic hazards. The area was overpopulated because subsistence farming did not allow demographic growth; it therefore became an area of high out-migration, especially towards Dakar and France (Lericollais 1975; 1981). The 1970-1989 period was particularly difficult, and marked by repeated droughts in 1972-1974 and 1983-1984, which probably explains the stagnation of children's anthropometry observed between 1957 and 1993.

The situation changed in the late 1980s when a real agricultural revolution occurred. Two dams on the river were built: Diama (1986) downstream, and Manantali (1990) upstream. Irrigated cultivation developed a lot, becoming preponderant after 1990, with more than 40,000 ha of irrigated land in 1990. New crops were introduced, in particular rice and onions, allowing better nutrition and an increase in farmers' income. Agricultural techniques were improved, as was the organization of agricultural production (Crousse et al. 1991; Le Roy 2006). In addition, remittances from emigrants increased significantly. These recent developments probably contributed to the improvement of the nutritional situation since 1990. To this, one should add major improvements in the control of infectious diseases, clearly visible in the impressive drop in under-five mortality which, according to DHS surveys, went from 200 per 1000 in 1986 to 54 per 1000 in 2018 in the River valley. In fact, infectious diseases control is one of the main factors of children' stunting and retarded growth.

DISCUSSION

The MISOES survey retains its full value, even long after, because it is the only quantitative benchmark of children's nutritional status in this region before independence (1960). In addition, the survey covers children of all ages up to 12 years, while most subsequent surveys covered only children under the age of 5 years. Furthermore, the MISOES data appeared very consistent with American standards, and therefore appear to be particularly precise and reliable.

The MISOES survey found a fairly good diet for the population of the valley, with an adequate caloric ration, sufficient intakes of proteins, lipids, minerals (iron), and vitamins. The only notable deficits were an insufficient intake of Vitamin A (80% of the needs) and of Vitamin C (58% of the needs) (Boutillier, Cantrelle et al. 1962). However, the population was subject to a high prevalence of infectious diseases, as shown by the high mortality of children. In addition, especially in rural areas, many children aged 8 and over were already at work, not going to school, and exercising a fairly intense physical activity, which can lead to low fat mass, while maintaining muscular mass.

On the whole, anthropometric deficits appeared clearly in all comparisons made with American references, and were often significant, even in small 2-year age groups. Two groups were particularly at high risk: the 1-2 year olds, a typical age group of protein-energy malnutrition, and the 9-12 year olds, the pre-adolescent age, an age group that is less studied. This last group appears to be particularly vulnerable for most of the indicators selected, and in particular for fat mass (skinfolds deficits).

Gender differences appeared small in general, and probably negligible before 8 years of age. However, the strong deficit of pre-adolescent boys and girls (9-12 years) in skinfolds can be a handicap and in particular can delay puberty. This observation could be related to the age at first menstruation (data not available in the MISOES survey). The smaller hip width for pre-adolescent girls could also have implications for deliveries, especially for girls who deliver before age 18, a frequent occurrence in this area.

Differences by place of residence were somewhat more pronounced. These are complex differences, not a universal comparative advantage from one environment over the other one, for anthropometric indicators as well as for other indicators available in the MISOES survey. The nutritional status measured by anthropometry is the result of diet, infections, physical exercise and the genetic endowment inherited from the parents. Infections appeared more prevalent in rural areas, while mortality was slightly higher in urban areas. Skinfolds were weaker in rural areas, but arm and muscle circumferences were weaker in urban areas. This apparent conundrum could be due to nutritional differences as well as to physical exercise. It appears that children in rural areas had a slightly lower fat mass, but a slightly higher muscle mass, which could contribute to the mortality differential. This study deserves to be continued, and in particular the apparent urban penalty, marked by a slight excess mortality and a slightly lower nutritional status. Have these differences noted in 1957 persisted?

The study of children's morphology shows that deficits in skeletal development were widespread, even at equal height. The ratios of shoulder and hips to stature were unfavorable, even if the acromio-iliac ratio was approximately retained. This shows that nutritional deficits were deep and affected the entire skeleton. The favorable leg length is probably due to a genetic characteristic, which is also found in all Sahelian populations.

The differences with the Niakhar area should be interpreted with caution. First, they are more than a quarter of a century apart, and it is possible that the observed gradient could have been reversed if the two nutritional surveys had been conducted at the same time. Indeed, in 1957 infant and child mortality in Niakhar was significantly higher (434 per 1,000) than in the river region, and the nutritional status was probably lower than it was in 1983-1984.

Put into perspective with recent data from the DHS surveys (1993-2017), the most recent of which being conducted 60 years after the MISOES survey, results indicate that for a long time the nutritional status of children in the valley had not improved, and that it changed only recently. This gives even greater value to the MISOES data. Why has anthropometry of under-five children stagnated for 35 years, when the mortality of these children was reduced? Why did the children start to grow while the weight did not follow? These open questions deserve special attention from nutritionists, demographers, economists and all development specialists.

REFERENCES

Boutillier JL, Cantrelle P, Causse J, Laurent C, N'Doye Th. (1962). *La moyenne vallée du Sénégal. Étude socio-économique.* Paris, INSEE, Service de la Coopération, 395 p. [*The middle valley of Senegal. Socio-economic study.*]

Cantrelle P. (1969). Étude démographique dans la région du Sine-Saloum (Sénégal): État civil et observation démographique, 1963-1965. *Travaux et Documents de l'O.R.S.T.O.M.*, no 1, Paris: ORSTOM. [Demographic study in the region of Sine-Saloum (Senegal): Civil status and demographic observation, 1963-1965. *Works and Documents of the O.R.S.T.O.M.*]

Crousse B, Mathieu P, Seck SM. (eds.). (1991). *La vallée du fleuve Sénégal: évaluations et perspectives d'une décennie d'aménagements (1980-1990).* Paris, France, Karthala, 380 p. [*The Senegal river valley: evaluations and perspectives of a decade of development*]

Centers for Disease Control. (2000). CDC Growth Charts for the United States: Methods and Development. 2000: *CDC Series Report 11*, No. 246, 201 pp.

Garenne M, Cantrelle P, Diop I.L. (1985). Le cas du Sénégal. In: Vallin J., Lopez A. (eds.). *La lutte contre la mort. Influence des politiques sociales et des politiques de santé sur l'évolution future de la mortalité.* Paris: PUF, pp 307-329. [*The fight against death. Influence of social policies and health policies on the future evolution of mortality.*]

Garenne M, Cantrelle P. (1989). Prospective studies of communities: their unique potential for studying the health transition. Reflections from the ORSTOM experience in Senegal. In: John Cleland and Allan Hill (eds.). *The Health Transition: Methods and Measures.* Proceedings of an International Workshop, London 7-9 June, 1989. pp 251-258.

Garenne M, Cantrelle P. (1997). Three decades of research on population and health: the ORSTOM experience in rural Senegal: 1962-1991. In: Das Gupta M., Garenne M. (eds.), *Prospective community studies in developing countries.* Oxford (UK): Oxford University Press, pp. 233-252.

Garenne M, Cantrelle P, Delaunay V, Becker C, Douillot L, Dione D, Diallo A, Sokhna C. (2018). Cinquante ans de transition de la mortalité à Niakhar (1963-2012). In: Delaunay V., Desclaux A., Sokhna C. (eds.). *Niakhar, mémoires et perspectives. Recherches pluridisciplinaires sur le changement en Afrique.* Marseille: Éditions de l'IRD et Dakar: L'Harmattan Sénégal. Chapitre 7, pp. 151-170, [Fifty years of mortality transition in Niakhar (1963-2012). In: Delaunay V., Desclaux A., Sokhna C. (eds.). *Niakhar, memories and perspectives. Multidisciplinary research on change in Africa*]

Garenne M, Maire B, Fontaine O, Dieng K, Briend A. (2000). Risques de décès associés à différents états nutritionnels chez l'enfant d'âge préscolaire. *Études du CEPED* n° 17, Paris CEPED, 192 p. [Risks of Death Associated with Different Nutritional States in Preschool Children. *CEPED studies n° 17*]

Garenne M. (2018). Tendances de l'état nutritionnel des jeunes enfants dans les pays francophones du Sahel: 1990-2015. *Ferdi, Document de travail P245.* [Trends in the nutritional status of young children in Francophone Sahelian countries: 1990-2015. *Ferdi, Working Paper P245.*]

Garenne M. (2020). Taller but thinner: Trends in child anthropometry in Senegal, 1990-2015. *Public Heath Nutrition.* (epublished January 3, 2020)

Groupe de Démographie Africaine. (1973a). *Sources et analyses des données démographiques. Application à l'Afrique d'expression française et à Madagascar. Tome 1: Source des données.* Paris, Ministère de la Coopération. [*Sources and analyzes of demographic data. Application to French-speaking Africa and Madagascar. Volume 1: Data source*]

Groupe de Démographie Africaine. (1973b). *Sources et analyses des données démographiques. Application à l'Afrique d'expression française et à Madagascar. Tome 2: Ajustement des données imparfaites.* Paris, Ministère de la Coopération. [*Sources and analyzes of demographic data. Application to French-speaking Africa and Madagascar. Volume 2: Adjusting imperfect data*]

Groupe de Démographie Africaine. (1977). *Sources et analyses des données démographiques. Application à l'Afrique d'expression française et à Madagascar. Tome 3: Analyse des données.* Paris, Ministère de la Coopération. [*Sources and analyzes of demographic data. Application to French-speaking Africa and Madagascar. Volume 3: Data Analysis*]

Lericollais A. (1975). Peuplement et migrations dans la vallée du Sénégal. *Cahiers ORSTOM, Série Sciences Humaines*; 13(2) : 123-135. [Settlement and migration in the Senegal valley. ORSTOM Notebooks, *Human Sciences Series*]

Lericollais A. (1981). La vallée du Sénégal. *Études Scientifiques*; (déc. 1981/12): 5-13. [The Senegal valley. *Scientific studies*]

Le Roy X. (2006). Agriculture irriguée et inégalités sociales dans la vallée du fleuve Sénégal. *PCSI - 4e Séminaire international et interdisciplinaire*, CIRAD, Montpellier, France. 13 p. (cirad-00153767). [Irrigated agriculture and social inequalities in the Senegal river valley. *PCSI - 4th International and Interdisciplinary Seminar*, CIRAD, Montpellier, France.]

National Center for Health Statistics (NCHS). (1996). *Third National Health and Nutrition Examination Survey (NHANES III), 1988-94.* U.S. Department of Health and Human Services (DHHS), Hyattsville, MD.

Chapter 3

OBESITY AND ANTHROPOMETRY

Archana Khanna, PhD*
Assistant Professor, Department of Physiotherapy, School of Allied Health Sciences, Sharda University, Greater Noida, Uttar Pradesh, India

ABSTRACT

Overweight and obesity are associated with an increased risk of cardiovascular disease and considered to be one of the leading risk factors for mortality. Numerous health risks are associated with different types of fat distribution patterns. It has been found that central obesity is associated with a number of metabolic abnormalities such as hypertension, hyperinsulinemia, and hyperlipidemia. Anthropometry is a science which deals with the measurements of human size, shape and proportion. It encompasses a variety of human body measurements such as weight, stature, skinfold thickness, circumferences, limb lengths, and breadths. Various anthropometric methods are available for the assessment of body fat. The general and central obesity anthropometric measures used for assessing adiposity-related risk include body mass index, waist circumference, hip circumference, waist-to-hip ratio, waist-to-stature ratio and body adiposity index. Central obesity measures including waist circumference and waist-hip ratio are considered better

---

* Corresponding Author's E-mail: archana.khanna@sharda.ac.in.

markers of the risk of Coronary Heart Disease (CHD) than body mass index among obese people. Fat distribution determines the cardio-metabolic problems associated with adiposity rather than total body fat. This can be due to an imbalance in the production of inflammatory and anti-inflammatory adipokines. Anthropometric measurements are among the simplest, non-invasive and low-cost methods to measure obesity and the risk of CHD among mass populations. The present chapter deals with the various methods used for assessing body fat and their application for obese individuals to predict the risk of CHD.

Keywords: obesity, anthropometry, waist to hip ratio, BMI, cardiovascular disease

1. INTRODUCTION

The World Health Organization (WHO) defines obesity as abnormal or excessive fat accumulation that may impair health [1]. The high prevalence of obesity has become a major global health challenge, since obesity is associated with severe health consequences, contributing to the increase in cardiovascular morbidity and mortality [2, 3]. It was estimated by the World Health Organization (WHO) that in 2016 more than 1.9 billion adults were overweight and over 650 million people suffered from obesity [4]. Obesity is an important risk factor for heart diseases and exerts adverse effects on cardiovascular function and structure.

Positive relationships between CVD mortality and BMI have been observed in a number of studies [5].

The fat distribution is affected by a number of factors including race, gender, age, genetic components, and lifestyle [7]. Type II and type III obesity are often called the central obesity and women are more likely to develop gynoid-type obesity [8]. Different types of obesity [9] can be described as follows:

- Type I obesity: It is characterized by excess body mass or percentage of fat without any particular concentration of fat in a given area of the body

- Type II obesity: It is characterized by excess subcutaneous fat on the trunk, particularly in the abdominal area (android or apple-shaped obesity)
- Type III obesity: It is characterized by excess abdominal visceral fat
- Type IV obesity: It is characterized by excess fat on the truncal-abdominal or the gluteo- femoral area (gynoid or pear-shaped obesity)

Table 1. Classification of overweight and obesity by BMI, waist circumference, and associated disease risk [6]

	BMI (kg/m^2)	Obesity Class	Disease Risk (Relative to Normal Weight and Waist Circumference)	
			Men ≤ 40 inches (≤ 102 cm) Women ≤ 35 inches (≤ 88 cm)	> 40 in (> 102 cm) > 35 in (> 88 cm)
Underweight	< 18.5		-	-
Normal	18.5–24.9		-	-
Overweight	25.0–29.9		Increased	High
Obesity	30.0–34.9	I	High	Very High
	35.0–39.9	II	Very High	Very High
Extreme Obesity	≥ 40	III	Extremely High	Extremely High

Numerous health risks are associated with different types of fat distribution patterns. Central obesity is associated with a number of metabolic abnormalities such as hypertension, hyperinsulinemia, and hyperlipidemia [10, 11]. Hence, there is an increased risk of developing cardiovascular diseases [11], and metabolic syndrome [12]. Due to high prevalence of obesity, it has become a major global health challenge and found to be associated with severe health consequences, contributing to the increase in cardiovascular morbidity and mortality [13, 3].

The greater amount of trunk or abdominal fat in comparison to hips and lower limbs has been found to be associated with an increased risk for hypertension, type 2 diabetes mellitus, and heart disease among both men and women [14, 15]. However, the relationships between central adiposity with co-morbidities vary by race and ethnicity. For example, in Asian descent population, abdominal (central) obesity has been identified to be a better disease risk predictor, especially for type 2 diabetes, than BMI [16].

Anthropometry is a science which deals with the measurements of body and those body parts which are related to kinetics and kinematics. Anthropometry is derived from Greek words, "Anthropos" meaning human and "Meteron" meaning measure. Anthropometry involves multiple human body measurements. Weight, stature (standing height), recumbent length, skinfold thicknesses, circumferences (head, waist, limb, etc.), limb lengths, and breadths (shoulder, wrist, etc.) are examples of anthropometric measures. These measurements are non-invasive and inexpensive to assess patients' nutritional status and have been used widely in clinical practice. A number of anthropometric methods are used to measure body fat also. These include body mass index (BMI), waist circumference (WC), hip circumference (HC), waist-to-hip ratio (WHR), waist-to-stature ratio (WSR) and body adiposity index (BAI) [17].

1.1. BMI

Body mass index or BMI is weight in kilograms divided by square of height in meters. BMI has been used extensively to identify and classify obesity. It is suggested as an ideal measure of adiposity since it is easy to measure and closely associated with obesity related health risks [18]. However, BMI cannot reflect the amount and distribution of body fat or clearly distinguish fat free mass from fat mass compartment. BMI performance in severely obese patients is impaired due to the large amount of subcutaneous adipose tissue and oedema [19, 20]. A given BMI may not correspond to the same proportion of body fat in different persons or populations [21, 22]. At a given BMI, Asians have significantly higher percentage body fat content as compared to whites and blacks [21]. It has been reported that Hispanic Americans in United States with a BMI < 30 are likely to have more body fat than African Americans and white Americans with the same BMI [22]. BMI is very useful to monitor the treatment of obesity, with a weight change of about 3.5 kg needed to produce a unit change in BMI. In adults, BMI levels above 25 are associated with an increased risk of morbidity and mortality, [23] with BMI levels of 30 and greater indicating obesity [24].

1.2. Circumference

It measures the size of a given body region that is composed of bone, lean, adipose, and residual tissues. It is assumed that at a constant thickness of skin and subcutaneous adipose tissue thickness around lean tissues, a greater circumference for individuals of the same body size indicates a greater visceral adipose tissue/lean tissue development. Common sites of circumference measurement include the mid-upper arm circumference and waist circumference.

1.2.1. Arm Circumference

Mid-upper arm circumference (MUAC) is a well-known anthropometric measurement as a marker of nutritional status in children or pregnant women. The measurement is easy to perform using simple and fewer apparatus. It can be measured easily on the debilitated individuals also. Being independent of height, it indicates the arm muscle and subcutaneous fat. MUAC has potential as an accurate, simple and widely available indicator of overweight and obesity in children and adolescents [25].

1.2.2. Waist Circumference

Waist and abdominal circumferences are frequently used to measure central obesity and visceral fat accumulation. Waist circumference measurement is a widely adopted method owing to its simplicity as compared to other methods that require measurements at multiple sites. It is measured with a non-stretchable tape to the nearest 0.1 cm, in a standing position during end-tidal expiration at the midpoint of the lowest rib cage and the iliac crest [26]. Cardiovascular disease risk based on waist circumference are given as ≥ 102 cm in men and ≥ 88 cm in women [27]. Among north Indian population, several waist circumference cut-off points were evaluated in relation to BMI cut-off points and cardiovascular diseases. The proposed action level for adult Asian Indians was set as: action level 1: men, ≥ 78 cm, women, ≥ 72 cm; and action level 2: men, ≥ 90 cm, women, ≥ 80 cm [28]. Waist circumference is more strongly associated with abdominal subcutaneous adipose tissue rather than visceral adipose tissue (VAT) [29]. Waist circumference has been found to be a key risk factor for metabolic abnormalities and development of chronic diseases. [30, 31].

1.3. Skinfold Measurements

Skinfold measurement is useful for assessment of subcutaneous fat distribution pattern. It is a measure of subcutaneous fat thickness at various regions of the body, by estimating body density and using it in equations to derive percent body fat. It was first used by Czech anthropologist Jindřich Matiegka in 1921 [32] and considered as a non-invasive, portable, and cost-effective approach that provides indication of both regional and overall subcutaneous fatness. The commonly used calipers are Holtain, Lange and Harpenden, which measure to the nearest 0.2 mm. The skinfold calipers have limited utility in the overweight or obese adult, the primary limitation being that most of them have an upper measurement limit of 45 to 55 mm, which restricts their use to subjects who are moderately overweight or thinner. Measurements are usually taken at sites such as biceps, triceps, subscapular and suprailiac, which are then used in age- and gender-specific equations, to arrive at values of body density [33]. Body fat is obtained from body density using a population specific conversion formula [34]. The estimates of percent body fat and fat free mass from skinfold method were found to be accurate in Indian adults when hydrodensitometry (HD) was used as reference [35]. However, when body fat mass estimates from skinfold methods were compared with the 4 compartment method, the mean error was found to be 6.6 kg in a group of south Indian adults [36].

1.4. Waist-Hip Ratio

The waist-hip ratio (WHR) is a measure of lower and upper body fat distribution and measures the storage of body fat. WHR is calculated by dividing the waist circumference by the hip circumference and the indicators of cardiovascular disease risk are ≥ 1.0 for men and ≥ 0.85 for women [27]. Android or excess upper body fat is seen more typically in men, while gynoid or excess lower body fat is seen more in women. It has been suggested that a high waist to hip ratio indicates an increased risk of obesity-related health conditions. However, as the level of fatness increases, the accuracy of waist to hip ratio to assess visceral fat decreases.

1.5. Bioelectrical Impedance Analysis (BIA)

Bioelectrical impedance analysis technique is used to predict body composition based, on the electrical conductive properties of the body [37]. BIA works on the principle that lean body mass (composed of water and electrolytes) is a good electrical conductor in comparison to the body fat which is a poor conductor. Using this method, total body water (TBW), fat-free mass (FFM), and fat mass can be estimated. It is achieved by measuring the resistance of the body as a conductor to a very small alternating electrical current [38, 39]. The BIA device can be single frequency (at 50 kHz), or multifrequency, when a wide range of frequencies are used.

Using multifrequency BIA, total body water can be divided into intracellular water (ICW) and extracellular water (ECW) compartments

[40]. BIS can also provide estimates of body cell mass (BCM) by differentiating between ECW and ICF spaces [40]. Numerous factors such as limb length, physical activity, nutrition status, hydration level, and placement of electrodes can be a source of error in BIA [41]. BIA provides quick, easy and relatively inexpensive estimates of FFM and TBW in healthy populations and in obese individuals, provided standardized methods and instruments are used. Being a portable, safe and easy to use instrument with low cost, it is a useful tool.

2. APPLICATIONS OF ANTHROPOMETRIC MEASUREMENTS IN OBESITY

Anthropometric measurements have been used to measure body fat. Cardiovascular disease risk has been found to be associated with both general and central obesity [42-48]. General and central obesity anthropometric measures for assessing adiposity-related risk include body mass index (BMI), waist circumference (WC), hip circumference (HC), waist-to-hip ratio (WHR), waist-to-stature ratio (WSR) and body adiposity index (BAI).

Borch et al., assessed the impact of various obesity measures on identification of subjects at risk and their respective risk estimates for venous thromboembolism. BMI, waist circumference, hip circumference and waist hip ratio was measured in 6708 subjects aged 25-84 years. It was concluded that waist circumference is the preferable anthropometric measure of obesity to identify subjects at risk for venous thromboembolism [49].

Pelegrini et al., found that all anthropometric indicators were able to diagnose excess body fat. However, BMI, waist to hip ratio and waist circumference had greater ability to discriminate body fat in both genders compared to the C-Index. They found that not only indicators of general obesity (BMI), but also indicators of central obesity (WC, WHtR) can be used in adolescents to diagnose high body fat [50].

Golia et al., conducted a study on 300 CHD patients and 100 age and sex-matched healthy controls, aged 45-70 years. Anthropometric measurements for waist and hip circumference, waist hip ratio, body mass index, and body fat percentage were taken to assess the prevalence of obesity among the selected population. A uniform distribution of waist circumference (WC), waist-hip ratio (WHR), and visceral fat percentage among patients of both sexes was observed. These were also found to be stronger predictors of risk of CHD relative to the BMI [51].

Dirani et al., conducted a study to investigate the relationship between anthropometric parameters and diabetic retinopathy in 500 adults with diabetes. Anthropometric measures included height, weight, BMI, waist, hip, neck and head circumferences and skinfold measurements. It was concluded that diabetics with higher BMI and larger neck circumference were more likely to have diabetic retinopathy and its severe stages. They also suggested obesity as an independent risk factor for diabetic retinopathy [52].

A systematic review conducted by Jayawardena et al., showed that novel anthropometric parameters had correlation with obesity and/or related metabolic risk factors [53].

Zhang et al., compared the predictive capability of direct and indirect adiposity measures in identifying people at risk of metabolic abnormalities. They measured height, body weight, waist and hip circumference, BMI, waist to hip ratio and waist to height ratio in 2780 women and 1160 men. It was found that in women, waist to hip ratio was best in identifying hypertension, dyslipidemia, hyperuricemia, diabetes and metabolic syndrome. It was concluded that waist to hip ratio was the best predictor of various metabolic abnormalities and BMI may be used as an alternative measure of obesity for identifying hypertension in both sexes [54].

Gaya et al., conducted a study to determine the association between cardiometabolic risk with body mass index and skinfold independently or in combination in youth aged 10 to 18 years old. It was found that overweight or obese individuals had the strongest association with cardiometabolic risk. Body mass index had the strongest association with cardiometabolic risk in comparison to skinfold thickness. [55].

Amirabdollahian and Haghighatdoost assessed prevalence of Metabolic Syndrome (MetS) in young adult population and made comparison between weight- and shape-oriented measures of adiposity. Healthy males and females aged 18–25 years from the Northwest of England were recruited using convenience sampling. BMI, waist circumference (WC), waist-to-height ratio (WHtR), waist-to-hip ratio (WHR), new BMI, Body Adiposity Index (BAI), Clinica Universidad de Navarra-Body Adiposity Estimator (CUN-BAE), and A Body Shape Index (ABSI) were assessed. Amongst all indices, the best predictor for cardiometabolic risk was WHtR, while ABSI had the weakest correlation with body fat, MetS, and cardiometabolic risk. Indices directly associated with WC and specifically WHtR had greater diagnostic power in detection of cardiometabolic risk in young adults [56].

Zhu et al., conducted a study to evaluate lipid profile distribution and to find the best anthropometric parameter associated with lipid disorders in children with obesity in 2243 school children aged 7–17 years. They concluded that the distribution of lipid profiles in Chinese children differed between younger and older age groups, and it fluctuated remarkably during 10 to 14 years. BMI had better practical utility in identifying dyslipidemia among school-aged children with obesity compared with other anthropometric measures [57].

Liu et al., aimed to compare the predictive value of a body shape Index with 5 conventional obesity-related anthropometric indices (body mass index, waist circumference, hip circumference, waist-to-hip ratio, waist-to-height ratio) in Chinese population and found waist-to-height ratio to be the best indicator for dyslipidemia, hyperglycemia, and CVDs. Waist circumference had a better prediction for abnormal blood pressure [58].

Luksiene et al., conducted a study to estimate trends in anthropometric indexes from 1992 to 2008 and to evaluate the risk of cardiovascular disease mortality in relation to anthropometric indexes. Body mass index, waist circumference, waist:hip ratio and waist:height ratio was found to be good indicators of cardiovascular disease mortality risk only in men aged 45–64 years [59].

Gilani et al., assessed the repeated measurements of body mass index (BMI), waist circumference (WC), waist to hip ratio (WHR) and waist to height ratio (WHtR) in predicting CHD incidence and concluded that WHtR is superior to other indices in predicting CHD incidence [60].

Zhang et al., determined the optimal cut-off values and evaluated the associations of body mass index (BMI), waist circumference (WC) and waist-height ratio (WHtR) with cardiovascular disease (CVD) risk factors. The survey was conducted among 35,256 adults aged 20–74 years in Shanghai. WHtR was found to be the best for discriminating hypertension and diabetes. They suggested it to be used as a standard screening tool in public health [61].

Goh et al., conducted a study to ascertain which anthropometric measurements of obesity, general or central, are better predictors of cardiovascular disease (CVD) risk in women. It was found that waist circumference (WC), waist-to-hip ratio (WHR) and waist-to-stature ratio had larger effects on increased CVD risk compared with body mass index (BMI). These central obesity measures also had higher sensitivity and specificity in identifying women above and below the 20% treatment threshold than BMI. Central obesity measures also recorded better correlations with CVD risk compared with general obesity measures. WC and WHR were found to be significant and independent predictors of CVD risk [62].

Tallon et al., conducted a study to describe Portuguese adolescents' anthropometric profile, Resting Metabolic Rate (RMR) and physical activity (PA) level and found that boys were significantly taller, heavier and had a significantly higher RMR than girls ($p < 0.01$). The overall prevalence of overweight/obesity was 16.5% and 5.9%, respectively. Only 38.3% of the participants were engaging in "moderate", "intense" or "very intense" physical activity and boys were more likely than girls to engage in these types of physical activity [63].

Kamadjeu et al., conducted a baseline survey in Cameroon to find prevalence and distribution of overweight and obesity using anthropometric measurements. They found high prevalence of overweight and obesity over 35 years of age especially among women [64].

Elisabeth et al., measured weight, height, BMI, arm circumference, average deltoid skinfold thickness, and average triceps skinfold thickness on 58 obese and severely obese Hispanic females aged 14 to 24 years. Significant differences were observed between the obese and severely obese groups for weight, BMI, arm circumference, and triceps skinfold thickness.

CONCLUSION

This chapter highlights the role of anthropometry in obesity. Anthropometric measurements including BMI, waist to hip ratio, waist circumference are one of the few methods that are used to estimate the level of body fat, hence obesity. Out of these measures, BMI, waist to hip ratio and waist circumference have been found to be the strong predictors of cardiovascular disease. These simple, non-invasive techniques can be applied with accuracy to predict the risk of cardiovascular disease among obese individuals. Owing to the utility and limitations of available anthropometric methods, any of the best-suited methods can be chosen to assess body composition, hence obesity and cardiovascular disease risk.

REFERENCES

[1] World Health Organization. *Obesity: preventing and managing the global epidemic.* 2000.

[2] Ng, M., Fleming, T., Robinson, M., Thomson, B., Graetz, N., Margono, C., et al., 2014. Global, regional, and national prevalence of overweight and obesity in children and adults during 1980–2013: a systematic analysis for the global burden of disease study 2013. *Lancet,* 384, 766–81.

[3] World Health Organization. 2009. *Global health risks: mortality and burden of disease attributable to selected major risks.* Geneva: World Health Organization.

[4] World Health Organization. 2018. *Fact sheet—obesity and overweight.* 2018.

[5] Valavanis, I. K., Mougiakakou, S. G., Grimaldi, K. A., et al., 2010. A multifactorial analysis of obesity as CVD risk factor: use of neural network-based methods in a nutrigenetics context. *BMC Bioinformatics*, 11, 453.

[6] Clinical Guidelines on the Identification, Evaluation, and Treatment of Overweight and Obesity in Adults--The Evidence Report. National Institutes of Health. 1998. *Obesity Research, 6 Suppl 2*, 51S–209S.

[7] Cornier, M. A., Després, J. P., Davis, N., Grossniklaus, D. A., Klein, S., Lamarche, B., Lopez-Jimenez, F., Rao, G., St-Onge, M. P., Towfighi, A., Poirier, P., American Heart Association Obesity Committee of the Council on Nutrition, Physical Activity and Metabolism, Council on Arteriosclerosis, Thrombosis and Vascular Biology, Council on Cardiovascular Disease in the Young, Council on Cardiovascular Radiology and Intervention, Council on Cardiovascular Nursing, Council on Epidemiology and Prevention, & Council on the Kidney in Cardiovascular Disease, and Stroke Council. 2011. Assessing adiposity: a scientific statement from the American Heart Association. *Circulation, 124*(18), 1996–2019.

[8] Lemieux, S., Prud'homme, D., Bouchard, C., Tremblay, A., Després, J. P. 1993. Sex differences in the relation of visceral adipose tissue accumulation to total body fatness. *The American journal of clinical nutrition, 58*(4), 463–467.

[9] Bouchard, C. 1991. Heredity and the path to overweight and obesity. *Medicine and Science in Sports and Exercise,* 23(3):285–291.

[10] Rasouli, N., Molavi, B., Elbein, S. C., Kern, P. A. 2007. Ectopic fat accumulation and metabolic syndrome. *Diabetes, Obesity and Metabolism*, 9(1), 1–10.

[11] Arsenault, B. J., Beaumont, E. P., Després, J. P., & Larose, E. (2012). Mapping body fat distribution: a key step towards the identification of the vulnerable patient? *Annals of Medicine*, *44*(8), 758–772.

[12] International Diabetes Federation. 2007. *The IDF consensus definition of the metabolic syndrome in children and adolescents.* IDF, Brussels.

[13] Khaodhiar, L., McCowen, K. C., Blackburn, G. L. 1999. Obesity and its comorbid conditions. *Clinical Cornerstone*, *2*(3), 17–31.

[14] Janssen, I., Katzmarzyk, P. T., & Ross, R. (2004). Waist circumference and not body mass index explains obesity-related health risk. *The American Journal of Clinical Nutrition*, *79*(3), 379–384.

[15] Balkau, B., Deanfield, J. E., Després, J. P., Bassand, J. P., Fox, K. A., Smith, S. C., Jr, Barter, P., Tan, C. E., Van Gaal, L., Wittchen, H. U., Massien, C., Haffner, S. M. 2007. International Day for the Evaluation of Abdominal Obesity (IDEA): a study of waist circumference, cardiovascular disease, and diabetes mellitus in 168,000 primary care patients in 63 countries. *Circulation*, *116*(17), 1942–1951.

[16] Fujimoto, W. Y., Bergstrom, R. W., Boyko, E. J., Leonetti, D. L., Newell-Morris, L. L., & Wahl, P. W. 1995. Susceptibility to development of central adiposity among populations. *Obesity Research*, *3 Suppl. 2*, 179S–186S.

[17] Duren, D. L., Sherwood, R. J., Czerwinski, S. A., Lee, M., Choh, A. C., Siervogel, R. M., & Cameron Chumlea, W. (2008). Body composition methods: comparisons and interpretation. *Journal of diabetes science and technology*, *2*(6), 1139–1146.

[18] Wang, Y. 2004. Epidemiology of childhood obesity—methodological aspects and guidelines: what is new? *International Journal of Obesity* 28, S21–S28.

[19] Das, S. K. 2005. Body composition measurement in severe obesity. *Current opinion in clinical nutrition and metabolic care*, *8*(6), 602–606.

[20] Beechy, L., Galpern, J., Petrone, A., & Das, S. K. 2012. Assessment tools in obesity - psychological measures, diet, activity, and body composition. *Physiology and Behavior*, 107(1), 154–171.

[21] Deurenberg, P., Yap, M., & van Staveren, W. A. (1998). Body mass index and percent body fat: a meta analysis among different ethnic groups. *International journal of obesity and related metabolic disorders : journal of the International Association for the Study of Obesity*, 22(12), 1164–1171.

[22] Fernández, J. R., Heo, M., Heymsfield, S. B., Pierson, R. N., Jr, Pi-Sunyer, F. X., Wang, Z. M., Wang, J., Hayes, M., Allison, D. B., & Gallagher, D. (2003). Is percentage body fat differentially related to body mass index in Hispanic Americans, African Americans, and European Americans? *The American Journal of Clinical Nutrition*, 77(1), 71–75.

[23] WHO Obesity: preventing and managing the global epidemic. 1998. Geneva, *World Health Organization Programme of Nutr.* 6-3-1997.

[24] Chumlea, W. M. and Guo, S. 2000. Assessment and prevalence of obesity: application of new methods to a major problem. *Endocrine*, 13(2),135-42.

[25] Jaiswal, M., Bansal, R., Agarwal, A. (2017). Role of Mid-Upper Arm Circumference for Determining Overweight and Obesity in Children and Adolescents. *Journal of Clinical and Diagnostic Research: JCDR*, 11(8), SC05–SC08.

[26] WHO Expert Committee on Physical Status: the Use and Interpretation of Anthropometry (1993: Geneva, Switzerland) & World Health Organization. 1995. *Physical status: the use of and interpretation of anthropometry, report of a WHO expert committee.* World Health Organization.

[27] World Health Organization. *Obesity, prevention and managing the global epidemic.* Report of a WHO consultation on obesity. Geneva: WHO; 1998.

[28] Misra, A., Vikram, N. K., Gupta, R., Pandey, R. M., Wasir, J. S., Gupta, V. P. 2006. Waist circumference cutoff points and action

levels for Asian Indians for identification of abdominal obesity. *International Journal of Obesity*, 30(1), 106–111.

[29] Bosy-Westphal, A., Booke, C. A., Blöcker, T., Kossel, E., Goele, K., Later, W., Hitze, B., Heller, M., Glüer, C. C., & Müller, M. J. 2010. Measurement site for waist circumference affects its accuracy as an index of visceral and abdominal subcutaneous fat in a Caucasian population. *The Journal of Nutrition*, 140(5), 954–961.

[30] Benfield, L. L., Fox, K. R., Peters, D. M., Blake, H., Rogers, I., Grant, C., & Ness, A. 2008. Magnetic resonance imaging of abdominal adiposity in a large cohort of British children. *International journal of Obesity, 32*(1), 91–99.

[31] Berentzen, T. L., Ängquist, L., Kotronen, A., Borra, R., Yki-Järvinen, H., Iozzo, P., Parkkola, R., Nuutila, P., Ross, R., Allison, D. B., Heymsfield, S. B., Overvad, K., Sørensen, T. I., & Jakobsen, M. U. 2012. Waist circumference adjusted for body mass index and intra-abdominal fat mass. *PloS one*, 7(2), e32213.

[32] Brozek, J. and Prokopec, M. 2001. Historical note: early history of the anthropometry of body composition. *American Journal of Human Biology,* 13(2):157–158.

[33] Durnin, J. V., & Womersley, J. (1974). Body fat assessed from total body density and its estimation from skinfold thickness: measurements on 481 men and women aged from 16 to 72 years. *The British Journal of Nutrition*, 32(1), 77–97.

[34] Siri, W E. 1993. Body composition from fluid spaces and density: Analysis of methods 1961. *Nutrition, 9:* 480-91.

[35] Kuriyan, R., Petracchi, C., Ferro-Luzzi, A., Shetty, P. S., Kurpad, A. V. 1998. Validation of expedient methods for measuring body composition in Indian adults. *The Indian Journal of Medical Research*, 107, 37–45.

[36] Kuriyan, R., Thomas, T., Ashok, S., Jayakumar, J., Kurpad, A. V. 2014. A 4-compartment model based validation of air displacement plethysmography, dual energy X-ray absorptiometry, skinfold technique & bio-electrical impedance for measuring body fat in

Indian adults. *The Indian Journal of Medical Research*, *139*(5), 700–707.

[37] Khalil, S. F., Mohktar, M. S., Ibrahim, F. 2014. The theory and fundamentals of bioimpedance analysis in clinical status monitoring and diagnosis of diseases. *Sensors (Basel, Switzerland)*, 14(6), 10895–10928.

[38] Chumlea, W. C. and Guo, S. S. 1994. Bioelectrical impedance and body composition: present status and future directions. *Nutrition Reviews*, *52*(4), 123–131.

[39] Lukaski, H. C., Johnson, P. E., Bolonchuk, W. W., Lykken, G. I. 1985. Assessment of fat-free mass using bioelectrical impedance measurements of the human body. *The American Journal of Clinical Nutrition*, 41(4), 810–817.

[40] Lee, S. Y., and Gallagher, D. (2008). Assessment methods in human body composition. *Current Opinion in Clinical Nutrition and Metabolic Care*, *11*(5), 566–572.

[41] Bioelectrical impedance analysis in body composition measurement: National Institutes of Health Technology Assessment Conference Statement. 1996. *The American Journal of Clinical Nutrition*, 64(3), 524S–532S.

[42] Manson, J. E., Colditz, G. A., Stampfer, M. J., Willett, W. C., Rosner, B., Monson, R. R., Speizer, F. E., Hennekens, C. H. 1990. A prospective study of obesity and risk of coronary heart disease in women. *New England Journal of Medicine*, *322*(13), 882–889.

[43] Park, Y. S., and Kim, J. S. 2012. Obesity phenotype and coronary heart disease risk as estimated by the Framingham risk score. *Journal of Korean Medical Science*, 27(3), 243–249.

[44] Satoh, H., Kishi, R., Tsutsui, H. 2010. Body mass index can similarly predict the presence of multiple cardiovascular risk factors in middle-aged Japanese subjects as waist circumference. *Internal Medicine (Tokyo, Japan)*, 49(11), 977–982.

[45] Ryan, M. C., Fenster Farin, H. M., Abbasi, F., Reaven, G. M. 2008. Comparison of waist circumference versus body mass index in diagnosing metabolic syndrome and identifying apparently healthy

subjects at increased risk of cardiovascular disease. *The American Journal of Cardiology*, 102(1), 40–46.

[46] Ying, X., Song, Z. Y., Zhao, C. J., Jiang, Y. 2010. Body mass index, waist circumference, and cardiometabolic risk factors in young and middle-aged Chinese women. *Journal of Zhejiang University. Science. B*, 11(9), 639–646.

[47] Zhu, S., Heymsfield, S. B., Toyoshima, H., Wang, Z., Pietrobelli, A., Heshka, S. 2005. Race-ethnicity-specific waist circumference cutoffs for identifying cardiovascular disease risk factors. *The American Journal of Clinical Nutrition*, 81(2), 409–415.

[48] Huang, K. C., Lee, M. S., Lee, S. D., Chang, Y. H., Lin, Y. C., Tu, S. H., & Pan, W. H. (2005). Obesity in the elderly and its relationship with cardiovascular risk factors in Taiwan. *Obesity Research*, 13(1), 170–178.

[49] Borch, K. H., Braekkan, S. K., Mathiesen, E. B., Njølstad, I., Wilsgaard, T., Størmer, J., Hansen, J. B. 2010. Anthropometric measures of obesity and risk of venous thromboembolism: the Tromso study. *Arteriosclerosis, Thrombosis, and Vascular Biology*, 30(1), 121–127.

[50] Pelegrini, A., Silva, D. A., Silva, J. M., Grigollo, L., Petroski, E. L. 2015. Anthropometric indicators of obesity in the prediction of high body fat in adolescents. *Revista Paulista de Pediatria*, 33(1), 56-62.

[51] Golia, N., Krishan, K., & Kashyap, J. R. 2020. Assessment of Obesity by Using Various Anthropometric Measurements among Patients with Coronary Heart Disease Residing in North India. *Cureus*, 12(5), e7948.

[52] Dirani, M., Xie, J., Fenwick, E., Benarous, R., Rees, G., Wong, T. Y., Lamoureux, E. L. (2011). Are obesity and anthropometry risk factors for diabetic retinopathy? The diabetes management project. *Investigative Ophthalmology and visual science*, 52(7), 4416–4421.

[53] Jayawaradena, R., Ranasinghe, P., Ranathunga, T., Mathangasinghe, Y., Wasalathanththri, S., Hills, A. P. 2020. Novel anthropometric parameters to define obesity and obesity-related disease in adults: a systematic review. *Nutrition Reviews*, 78(6), 498-513.

[54] Zhang, Z. Q., Deng, J., He, L. P., Ling, W. H., Su, Y. X., and Chen, Y. M. 2013. Comparison of various anthropometric and body fat indices in identifying cardiometabolic disturbances in Chinese men and women. *PloS one*, 8(8), e70893.

[55] Gaya, A. R., Brand, C., Dias, A. F., Gaya, A., Lemes, V. B., & Mota, J. 2017. Obesity anthropometric indicators associated with cardiometabolic risk in Portuguese children and adolescents. *Preventive Medicine Reports*, 8, 158–162.

[56] Amirabdollahian, F., and Haghighatdoost, F. 2018. Anthropometric Indicators of Adiposity Related to Body Weight and Body Shape as Cardiometabolic Risk Predictors in British Young Adults: Superiority of Waist-to-Height Ratio. *Journal of Obesity*, 8370304.

[57] Zhu, Y., Shao, Z., Jing, J., Ma, J., Chen, Y., Li, X., Yang, W., Guo, L., Jin, Y. 2016. Body Mass Index Is Better than Other Anthropometric Indices for Identifying Dyslipidemia in Chinese Children with Obesity. *PloS one*, 11(3), e0149392.

[58] Liu, J., Tse, L. A., Liu, Z., Rangarajan, S., Hu, B., Yin, L., Leong, D. P., Li, W., and PURE (Prospective Urban Rural Epidemiology) study in China. 2019. Predictive Values of Anthropometric Measurements for Cardiometabolic Risk Factors and Cardiovascular Diseases Among 44 048 Chinese. *Journal of the American Heart Association*, 8(16), e010870.

[59] Luksiene, D., Tamosiunas, A., Virviciute, D., Bernotiene, G., Peasey, A. 2015. Anthropometric trends and the risk of cardiovascular disease mortality in a Lithuanian urban population aged 45-64 years. *Scandinavian Journal of Public Health*, 43(8), 882–889.

[60] Gilani, N., Kazemnejad, A., Zayeri, F., Hadaegh, F., Azizi, F., Khalili, D. 2017. Anthropometric Indices as Predictors of Coronary Heart Disease Risk: Joint Modeling of Longitudinal Measurements and Time to Event. *Iranian Journal of Public Health*, *46*(11), 1546–1554.

[61] Zhang, Y., Gu, Y., Wang, N. et al., 2019. Association between anthropometric indicators of obesity and cardiovascular risk factors among adults in Shanghai, China. *BMC Public Health,* 19, 1035.

[62] Goh, L. G., Dhaliwal, S. S., Welborn, T. A., Lee, A. H., and Della, P. R. 2014. Anthropometric measurements of general and central obesity and the prediction of cardiovascular disease risk in women: a cross-sectional study. *BMJ open*, 4(2), e004138.

[63] Tallon, J. M., Dias, S. R., Silva, A. J., Barros, A., Costa, A. M. 2019. Characterization of the anthropometric profile and physical activity levels of Portuguese adolescents. *Biometrics and Biostatistics International Journal*, 8(5),184-193.

[64] Kamadjeu, R. M., Edwards, R., Atanga, J. S., Kiawi, E. C., Unwin, N., Mbanya, J. C. 2006. Anthropometry measures and prevalence of obesity in the urban adult population of Cameroon: an update from the Cameroon Burden of Diabetes Baseline Survey. *BMC public health*, *6*, 228.

[65] Hastings, E. S., Anding, R. H., Middleman, A.B. 2011. Correlation of Anthropometric Measures Among Obese and Severely Obese Adolescents and Young Adults. *ICAN: Infant, Child, and Adolescent Nutrition*, 3(3), 171-174.

In: Anthropometry
Editor: Sébastien Legrand

ISBN: 978-1-53619-269-8
© 2021 Nova Science Publishers, Inc.

Chapter 4

THE EFFECT OF DIFFERENT TYPES OF EXERCISE ON ANTHROPOMETRIC MEASURES AND BODY COMPOSITION IN OLDER ADULTS

Pablo Monteagudo[*]
Department of Education and Specific Didactics,
Jaume I University, Castellon, Spain

ABSTRACT

Age-related changes regarding anthropometry or body composition such as the decrease in muscle mass, the increase in body fat, and the loss of bone mass have important systemic implications and are significant contributors to functional limitation in the old age. However, there is evidence supporting the positive role of physical exercise and active lifestyles in these variables.

---

[*] Corresponding Author's E-mail: pmonteag@uji.es.

The purpose of this chapter is to review the effect of different modalities of physical exercise on anthropometric measurements and body composition in different populations of older adults. Public health policies aimed to prescribe exercise programs must account for these specific implications.

INTRODUCTION

Physical exercise is becoming a key strategy for all health professionals and is starting to be considered both a basic and collective element that can turn around some inadequate lifestyles and unhealthy behaviors that are becoming more common (Vidarte-Claros et al. 2011). In fact, the American College of Sports Medicine (ACSM) has even stated that regular engagement in physical exercise is comparable to pharmacological treatment. Indeed, after confirming that physical activity promotes optimal health, it has become obvious that it is key to the prevention and treatment of many pathologies and should be included as part of regular medical care, and so the ACSM coined the catchphrase 'exercise is medicine.'

However, many people are not as physically active as they could be, and therefore the potential to maximize their health and well-being is diminished. As adults age, they tend to be less physically active, and as this decline in physical activity continues, the likelihood that older adults will be the least active population group increases (Hallal et al. 2012, McKee, Kearney, and Kenny 2015). According to the WHO, physical inactivity is among the top ten causes of death worldwide (WHO 2009) and it's one of the two top five health risk factors, along with obesity.

Given the above, the following chapter aims to summarize the main benefits produced by physical exercise in older adults—especially in relation to body composition—which have led it to become the backbone of every field of health, and therefore also of public health policies.

OBESITY AND OVERWEIGHT

The prevalence of overweight (a body mass index [BMI] of 25-29.9 kg/m2) and obesity (BMI > 30 kg/m2) has significantly increased over the last three decades, and concerns about the health risks associated with these problems have become almost global (Ng et al. 2014) because they now represent one of the main challenges to public healthcare providers. Physical inactivity is a major risk factor both for cardiovascular disease and for weight gain. Body fat accumulates when the energy content of the food and beverages consumed by an individual exceeds the energy expended by their metabolism and the physical activity they perform. Aging itself, together with family history, can lead to this energy imbalance. In addition, obesity places a higher cardiovascular and respiratory demand on individuals and can cause back and/or joint pain as a result of arthritis and the excess weight itself. Thus, weight gain can lead to decreased daily physical activity because individuals find it harder and more uncomfortable to engage in physical activity, thereby creating a negative feedback loop.

In this sense, there is strong scientific evidence based on long-term epidemiological studies that shows how physical activity helps people to maintain a stable body weight over time (Wareham, van Sluijs, and Ekelund 2005). However, physical activity alone is not entirely effective in reducing weight because a lot of activity is required, and so a reduction in calorie intake is also often required (Kallings et al. 2009, Street, Wells, and Hills 2015). Therefore, although nutritional control should be viewed with caution, joint strategies to achieve weight loss are often recommended.

In general, the issue of weight loss among older adults is a source of conflict, because if not carefully managed, it can have harmful consequences by increasing sarcopenia (loss of muscle mass) and decreasing bone mass. Therefore, it has been suggested that weight control in obese older adults should focus on maintaining muscle mass and improving physical function, rather than causing weight reduction per se. Randomized clinical trials conducted in obese older adults suggest that the combination of physical exercise with caloric restriction produces the greatest benefits in terms of physical function and quality of life (Rejeski et al. 2010). Furthermore, they also report positive changes in body composition such as decreased weight and fat mass, and better glycemic control (Dunstan et al. 2002, Rejeski et al. 2010).

In conclusion, the increased risk of mortality, cardiovascular disease, and functional impairment related to obesity can be considerably (although not completely) reduced by increasing physical activity, and this effect can be boosted even more if the aerobic physical condition of the individual is simultaneously improved (Fogelholm 2010, Koster et al. 2008). Therefore, promoting physical activity among obese senior citizens is highly recommended.

MUSCULOSKELETAL HEALTH

Musculoskeletal disorders are common among older adults and are the leading cause of functional limitations. However, physical activity has the potential to postpone or prevent these musculoskeletal disorders and can even contribute to rehabilitation and recovery after a period of post-surgical rest. Fractures, usually caused by falls, are another important and frequent problem among older adults, and these can be aggravated by the phenomenon known as osteoporosis—a reduction in bone mass and microarchitectural deterioration of bone tissues which increases bone fragility and therefore the risk of fractures.

Falls are a multifactorial problem that are not only affected by external risk factors (such as the environmental conditions at home and in the environment, the person's ease of local mobility, etc.), but also by internal factors such as low muscle strength, poor vision, or reduced mobility. Regularly engaging in physical activity helps to protect individuals from external stimuli as well as improving internal factors by, for example, improving their functional capacity, ability to concentrate, etc. Exercise can also reduce the risk of fractures by increasing bone strength and improving balance and mobility, thereby helping to prevent older people from falling and making them less susceptible to the effects of osteoporosis

(Bloomfield et al. 2004). Meta-analyzes of physical exercise interventions aimed at preserving bone mass suggest that programs for older adults should include not only cardiovascular endurance and/or strength activities (Kelley, Kelley, and Tran 2001, Martyn-St James and Carroll 2010), but also tasks designed to improve balance and prevent falls (Bloomfield et al. 2004) such as Tai-chi (Gillespie et al. 2012).

TRAINING PROGRAMS FOR OLDER ADULTS

A wide variety of training programs have been described for older adults. Within this range we can distinguish between exercises aimed at improving strength, cardiorespiratory fitness, balance, and the prevention of falls, or activities of a functional nature designed to improve gait speed, and generally maintain independence and autonomy. The type of exercise prescribed can be personalized within recommended guidelines, depending on the needs and interests of each individual. For example, aerobic training can be performed while walking, cycling, or swimming, but can also be trained through dance-based interventions, strength circuits with light loads, or sports activities such as Nordic walking or orientation, etc. which also simultaneously achieve improvements in other areas. Participating in various types of exercise or rotating between them to achieve the same physiological or functional benefit, can be a useful way to prevent boredom from interfering with long-term participation.

Therefore, it is important to choose the exercise type based on the physiological objective: in strength-resistance exercise programs designed to improve neuromuscular function, the loads are raised above the individual's threshold in short or intermittent sets to help improve their VO_2max, while these loads are lowered but delivered in longer sets when the aim is to improve cardiovascular function. Likewise, balance training stimulates improvements in proprioception thereby helping to prevent falls and positively influencing a multitude of other human motor skills (Martínez-Amat et al. 2013). However, programs designed to simultaneously improve several domains may be a more efficient means of achieving improvements in multiple physiological areas (Holviala et al. 2012).

In fact, multicomponent exercise programs that include strength, endurance, and balance training seem to lead to greater improvements than other types of intervention, because they simultaneously stimulate various components of physical health (Cadore et al. 2013). However, most community exercise programs or those based on ecological models (such as healthy walking programs) have been approached from a perspective oriented towards improving aerobic stamina (Brawley, Rejeski, and King 2003). For example, Patiño-Villena et al. (2016), carried out a community intervention (coordinated between the local government and the primary care center) based on professionally-guided neighborhood walks in urban areas which produced positive results in terms of cholesterol levels, hypertension, diabetes, stress, and body weight.

Thus, it seems that multicomponent programs at the clinical level, and programmed outings at the community level, have emerged as the main strategies to promote functional improvement among older adults. Thus, in the following sections we present a brief review of each of these programs, followed by a discussion of the conclusions reached by different studies in order to understand their reported effects on body composition and anthropometry in older adults.

Walking Based Training Programs

Because of its simplicity, the fact that no special equipment is required (making it inexpensive), and because it can be done alone or in company (usually within the local environment), walking is one of the key cardiovascular exercises prescribed to older people. In addition, this activity carries a low risk of injury and can be performed by frail senior citizens or those with moderate health problems such as cardiovascular disease (although support, adaptation, and monitoring by a movement professional is recommended in these cases). Furthermore, walking is most often selected by older adults as their physical activity of choice

(Gallagher, Clarke, and Carr 2016). For example, in Australia, walking was the most popular physical activity among people aged 45–54 and 55–64 (selected by 30% and 34%, respectively), compared to other exercise modalities (Australian New Zealand Society Geriatric Medicine 2014).

Several strategies are currently used to increase and maintain the participation of older people in walking programs. For instance, the use of pedometers and smart digital devices that record walking activity is becoming increasingly popular (Cavanaugh et al. 2007, Strath, Swartz, and Cashin 2009), although the acceptability of such instruments is subject to debate because their use may introduce an element of selectiveness depending on the groups who are able to or not able to use this type of technology. In addition, monitoring the number of steps taken during the day is just one form of physical activity recording; some older adults may prefer to count the number of minutes of activity they perform over the day or record the distance they walk, rather than use a device that counts their steps (Tudor-Locke et al. 2011).

Walking on a treadmill is another form of walking that some older adults may prefer, and so the availability of such a machine at home may be a good option for older adults who are not able to go outside for health or other reasons (Watt et al. 2010). Furthermore, these machines offer balance supports and have graduated intensity levels that can allow an older person to walk in a safe, climate-controlled environment. For senior citizens who want to socialize through exercise but would like to do so in a safe and climate-controlled environment, walking in a shopping center can also be a good option. However, compared to walking in the open air, mall walking may not be economical or offer so many opportunities for company or social support (Floegel et al. 2015).

Outdoor park-walking programs are becoming increasingly popular, as are some of the programs running in Australia, the United States, and Japan (COTA 2016, Farren et al. 2015, Kubota et al. 2020). Many of these programs are free and allow adults of any age range to participate in exercise in a safe, accessible, and affordable setting. Walking programs in public parks can include the possibility of warm-up exercises in structures for this sole purpose. They also usually create program leaders within groups of older adults who help to encourage participation (Farren et al. 2015). In other words, they have a strong social component which, along with the social and emotional benefits, improves adherence to the program. Thus, walking in groups has been shown to increase levels of exercise and so, leveraging the social benefits inherent in participation in a regular group activity could be a useful means to help older adults to maintain physical activity over time (Kassavou, Turner, and French 2013).

Likewise, walking interventions have been effective, for example, in increasing physical activity (Rosenberg et al. 2012), preventing cognitive decline (Maki et al. 2012), and in enhancing health-related quality of life (Awick et al. 2015) in healthy senior citizens. Furthermore, walking improves both functional and aerobic capacity, and reduces the risk of cardiovascular disease (Albright and Thompson 2006, Boone-Heinonen et al. 2009, Murtagh et al. 2015). However, its impact is less clear for sedentary older adults or those with mobility limitations (Rezola-Pardo et al. 2020).

Multicomponent Training Programs

Multicomponent training in older adults first emerged approximately a decade ago. These interventions combine tasks designed to work on strength, endurance, balance, flexibility, and coordination in the same session. In some cases, multicomponent programs have been developed that focus more attention on every aspect of one of these tasks, according to specific objectives such as, for example, increasing strength in older individuals with sarcopenia. Thus, we could define this type of program as the combination of aerobic and strength exercises, with cognitive, balance, and/or coordination tasks, with the aim of attaining comprehensive responses together with global physical activation (Bouaziz et al. 2016, Cadore et al. 2014, Toraman, Erman, and Agyar 2004).

Slowly but surely, data has emerged that has make it clear that this type of training improves body composition, functional capacity, executive function, and quality of life in older individuals (Forte et al. 2013, Marques et al. 2011, Nogueira et al. 2017, Wang et al. 2018). Likewise, Bouaziz et al. (2016) has discussed the positive effects this type of program has on respiratory fitness, neuromuscular function, and quality of life. A recent review of these programs by Marín-Cascales et al. (2018) showed that their effectiveness is greater when they are carried out for at least a year, even though improvements can appear after only 6 months. However, it is difficult to assess because the protocols used are not yet standardized and so there is a lot of heterogeneity regarding their design and in the training sessions themselves, for example, in terms of the exercise intensities and durations used. The benefits of this type of program have also been demonstrated in fragile senior citizens (Cadore et al. 2014). In addition, the role of the supervisor or coach in providing quality feedback to participants is especially important, especially among older age groups. Therefore, an important characteristic of these programs is that their participants receive instruction on the proper technique from qualified professionals (Bouaziz et al. 2016).

On the other hand, participation in multi-component programs is also associated with other advantages, such as improving long-term adherence among participants and favoring social interactions or creating a sense of mutual commitment among students. These scientific findings show the importance of encouraging older people to participate in multicomponent-style exercise programs, leading some authors to call for their more generalized implementation as part of current public health policies (Bouaziz et al. 2016).

EFFECTS OF BOTH TYPES OF EXERCISE ON BODY COMPOSITION

The benefits of the training programs described above in terms of body composition have been scientifically proven, although the type of exercise implemented seems to influence these benefits with respect to certain variables. On the one hand, Binder et al. (2005) did not achieve improvements (a reduction in the percentage of body fat) in sedentary and frail older adults after they had completed 6 months of a progressive strength-resistance program (3 days/week). In addition, Marques et al. (2009) found no differences in this variable after the completion of 8 months of exercise (2 days/week) by 2 different experimental groups—one on a strength program and the other on a multicomponent program. On the other hand, the improvements achieved in terms of reduced body fat percentage showed greater scientific consistency in aerobic-oriented walking programs (Beavers et al. 2017, Gába et al. 2016, Rosa et al. 2017).

However, both program types appeared to be effective at increasing muscle mass. Indeed, some longer-term studies have shown that multicomponent programs were able to increase muscle mass in postmenopausal women (Aragão et al. 2014) who trained 3 days/week for 12 months, i.e., longer and more frequent training than the programed schedule for the EFAM-UV© program (15 weeks and 2 sessions/week). However, given the heterogeneity of the protocols and training loads used, not all multicomponent programs seem to have the same effect on this variable (Marín-Cascales et al. 2018). Nonetheless, walking programs seem to show greater inconsistency in terms of increases in muscle mass, given that most studies fail to show any significant changes in this variable—at least at a more general level (Beavers et al. 2017, Gába et al. 2016, Karstoft et al. 2013).

Despite this, some authors have pointed out the importance of including aerobic exercise in multicomponent programs (Marín-Cascales et al. 2018). In this sense, walking is one of the most frequent forms of aerobic activity used in these programs. Therefore, the key to producing changes in muscle mass may be to integrate a volume of around 30 minutes of aerobic work alongside the other exercises (e.g., strength, agility, coordination, breathing) that make up the multicomponent programs (Marín-Cascales et al. 2018), thereby ensuring that all participants work at the correct intensity. In any case, even if an intervention does not produce increases in this variable, the results could be considered positive because they preserve muscle mass which in itself can potentially reduce the risk of death in older adults (Santanasto et al. 2017).

Finally, the results regarding the changes produced by these exercise modalities in terms of bone mass are somewhat less encouraging. Given the variability in the available protocols and the different measurement instruments presented in the bibliography, the results of these methods are difficult to quantify and compare (Benedetti et al. 2018). Most studies that have investigated the effect of aerobic walking programs on bone mass have not reported significant increases in this variable (Gómez-Cabello et al. 2012). Studies conducted with multicomponent interventions have not reported improvements in bone mass measured as bone mineral density (Marín-Cascales, Alcaraz, and Rubio-Arias 2017, Marques et al. 2011). Given all the above, maintaining or delaying the loss of bone mass in older adults should also be considered an important outcome of any physical exercise intervention for older adults.

Conclusion

In general terms, it seems that walking programs may cause increased body fat reduction in these populations and so, can be considered as an effective strategy to simultaneously improve cardiovascular function. The effects of training on muscle and bone mass reported in the literature remain disparate. Differences in parameters such as dose or intensity, as well as the complex biology involved in tissue homeostasis in these populations, could partly explain the inconsistency in these multicomponent training programs in terms of body composition outcomes in older adults.

It is important that both the administrations responsible for implementing prevention policies through physical exercise, as well as doctors—as essential agents in their prescription—clearly understand the impact of different strategies on body composition. Thus, to produce rapid changes in body composition and treat problems such as sarcopenia or dyslipidemia, aerobic programs could become a key element in the design of strategies to control weight in senior citizens, even though multicomponent programs are generally more beneficial, especially at the functional level. Finally, it is important to highlight the importance of supervised, periodic training by professionals specialized in physical exercise during aging as a means of maximizing its benefits by reducing the risk of obesity and the problems that can follow on from this pathology.

REFERENCES

Albright, Carolyn, and Dixie L Thompson. 2006. "The effectiveness of walking in preventing cardiovascular disease in women: a review of the current literature." *Journal of women's health* 15 (3):271-280.

Aragão, F, CG Abrantes, RE Gabriel, MF Sousa, C Castelo-Branco, and MH Moreira. 2014. "Effects of a 12-month multi-component exercise program on the body composition of postmenopausal women." *Climacteric* 17 (2):155-163. doi: 10.3109/13697137.2013.819328.

Awick, EA, TR Wójcicki, EA Olson, J Fanning, HD Chung, K Zuniga, M Mackenzie, AF Kramer, and E McAuley. 2015. "Differential exercise effects on quality of life and health-related quality of life in older adults: a randomized controlled trial." *Quality of Life Research* 24 (2):455-462.

Beavers, K. M., W. T. Ambrosius, W. J. Rejeski, J. H. Burdette, M. P. Walkup, J. L. Sheedy, B. A. Nesbit, J. E. Gaukstern, B. J. Nicklas, and A. P. Marsh. 2017. "Effect of Exercise Type during Intentional Weight Loss on Body Composition in Older Adults with Obesity." *Obesity (Silver Spring)* 25 (11):1823-1829. doi: 10.1002/oby.21977.

Benedetti, Maria Grazia, Giulia Furlini, Alessandro Zati, and Giulia Letizia Mauro. 2018. "The Effectiveness of Physical Exercise on Bone Density in Osteoporotic Patients." *BioMed research international* 2018.

Binder, Ellen F, Kevin E Yarasheski, Karen Steger-May, David R Sinacore, Marybeth Brown, Kenneth B Schechtman, and John O Holloszy. 2005. "Effects of progressive resistance training on body composition in frail older adults: results of a randomized, controlled trial." *The Journals of Gerontology Series A: Biological Sciences & Medical Sciences* 60 (11):1425-1431.

Bloomfield, Susan A, KD Little, ME Nelson, and VR Yingling. 2004. "American College of Sports Medicine position stand: physical activity and bone health." *Medicine Science in Sports Exercise* 195 (9131/04):3611.

Boone-Heinonen, Janne, Kelly R Evenson, Daniel R Taber, and Penny Gordon-Larsen. 2009. "Walking for prevention of cardiovascular disease in men and women: a systematic review of observational studies." *Obesity Reviews* 10 (2):204-217.

Bouaziz, W, PO Lang, E Schmitt, G Kaltenbach, B Geny, and T Vogel. 2016. "Health benefits of multicomponent training programmes in seniors: a systematic review." *International Journal of Clinical Practice* 70 (7):520-536. doi: 10.1111/ijcp.12822.

Brawley, Lawrence R, W Jack Rejeski, and Abby C King. 2003. "Promoting physical activity for older adults: the challenges for changing behavior." *American Journal of Preventive Medicine* 25 (3):172-183.

Cadore, E, Alvaro Casas-Herrero, Fabricio Zambom-Ferraresi, Fernando Idoate, Nora Millor, Marisol Gómez, Leocadio Rodriguez-Mañas, and Mikel Izquierdo. 2014. "Multicomponent exercises including muscle power training enhance muscle mass, power output, and functional outcomes in institutionalized frail nonagenarians." *Age and ageing* 36 (2):773-785.

Cadore, E, L Rodríguez-Mañas, A Sinclair, and M Izquierdo. 2013. "Effects of different exercise interventions on risk of falls, gait ability, and balance in physically frail older adults: a systematic review." *Rejuvenation Research* 16 (2):105-114.

Cavanaugh, James T, Kim L Coleman, Jean M Gaines, Linda Laing, and Miriam C Morey. 2007. "Using step activity monitoring to characterize ambulatory activity in community-dwelling older adults." *Journal of the American Geriatrics Society* 55 (1):120-124.

COTA. 2016. *Active Aging: Mall walking.* accessed 25/03/2019. http://www.cotawa.org.au/activeageing/mall-walking.

Dunstan, David W, Robin M Daly, Neville Owen, Damien Jolley, Maximilian De Courten, Jonathan Shaw, and Paul Zimmet. 2002. "High-intensity resistance training improves glycemic control in older patients with type 2 diabetes." *Diabetes Care* 25 (10):1729-1736.

Farren, Laura, Basia Belza, Peg Allen, Sarah Brolliar, David R Brown, Marc L Cormier, Sarah Janicek, Dina L Jones, Diane K King, and David X Marquez. 2015. "Peer Reviewed: Mall Walking Program Environments, Features, and Participants: A Scoping Review." *Preventing chronic disease* 12.

Floegel, TA, PR Giacobbi Jr, JM Dzierzewski, AT Aiken-Morgan, B Roberts, CS McCrae, M Marsiske, and MP Buman. 2015. "Intervention markers of physical activity maintenance in older adults." *American Journal of Health Behavior* 39 (4):487-499.

Fogelholm, Mikael. 2010. "Physical activity, fitness and fatness: relations to mortality, morbidity and disease risk factors. A systematic review." *Obesity reviews* 11 (3):202-221.

Forte, Roberta, Caterina Pesce, Joao Costa Leite, Giuseppe De Vito, Eileen R Gibney, Phillip D Tomporowski, and Colin AG Boreham. 2013. "Executive function moderates the role of muscular fitness in determining functional mobility in older adults." *Aging clinical experimental research* 25 (3):291-298.

Gába, Aleš, Roman Cuberek, Zdeněk Svoboda, František Chmelík, Jana Pelclová, Michal Lehnert, and Karel Frömel. 2016. "The effect of brisk walking on postural stability, bone mineral density, body weight and composition in women over 50 years with a sedentary occupation: a randomized controlled trial." *BMC women's health* 16 (1):63.

Gallagher, NA, P Clarke, and E Carr. 2016. "Physical activity in older adults in a combined functional circuit and walking program." *Geriatric Nursing* 37 (5):353-359. doi: 10.1016/j.gerinurse.2016.04.017.

Gillespie, Lesley D, M Clare Robertson, William J Gillespie, Catherine Sherrington, Simon Gates, Lindy M Clemson, and Sarah E Lamb.

2012. "Interventions for preventing falls in older people living in the community." *Cochrane database of systematic reviews* (9).

Gómez-Cabello, A, I Ara, A González-Agüero, J Casajus, and G Vicente-Rodriguez. 2012. "Effects of training on bone mass in older adults." *Journal of Sports Medicine* 42 (4):301-325. doi: 10.2165/11597670-000000000-00000.

Hallal, Pedro C, Lars Bo Andersen, Fiona C Bull, Regina Guthold, William Haskell, and Ulf Ekelund. 2012. "Global physical activity levels: surveillance progress, pitfalls, and prospects." *The lancet* 380 (9838):247-257.

Holviala, J, WJ Kraemer, E Sillanpää, H Karppinen, J Avela, A Kauhanen, A Häkkinen, and K Häkkinen. 2012. "Effects of strength, endurance and combined training on muscle strength, walking speed and dynamic balance in aging men." *European journal of applied physiology* 112 (4):1335-1347.

Kallings, Lena V, Justo Sierra Johnson, Rachel M Fisher, Ulf de Faire, Agneta Ståhle, Erik Hemmingsson, and Mai-Lis Hellénius. 2009. "Beneficial effects of individualized physical activity on prescription on body composition and cardiometabolic risk factors: results from a randomized controlled trial." *European Journal of Cardiovascular prevention and rehabilitation* 16 (1):80-84.

Karstoft, Kristian, Kamilla Winding, Sine H Knudsen, Jens S Nielsen, Carsten Thomsen, Bente K Pedersen, and Thomas P Solomon. 2013. "The effects of free-living interval-walking training on glycemic control, body composition, and physical fitness in type 2 diabetic patients: a randomized, controlled trial." *Diabetes care* 36 (2):228-236.

Kassavou, Aikaterini, Andrew Turner, and David P French. 2013. "Do interventions to promote walking in groups increase physical activity? A meta-analysis." *International Journal of Behavioral Nutrition Physical Activity* 10 (1):18.

Kelley, George A, Kristi S Kelley, and Zung Vu Tran. 2001. "Resistance training and bone mineral density in women: a meta-analysis of controlled trials." *American Journal of Physical Medicine & Rehabilitation* 80:65-77.

Koster, Annemarie, Kushang V Patel, Marjolein Visser, Jacques Th M Van Eijk, Alka M Kanaya, Nathalie De Rekeneire, Anne B Newman, Frances A Tylavsky, Stephen B Kritchevsky, and Tamara B Harris. 2008. "Joint effects of adiposity and physical activity on incident mobility limitation in older adults." *Journal of the American Geriatrics Society* 56 (4):636-643.

Kubota, Akio, Munehiro Matsushita, Takashi Arao, Dafna Merom, Ester Cerin, and Takemi Sugiyama. 2020. "A community-wide walking promotion using maps and events for Japanese older adults." *Journal of aging and health* 32 (7-8):735-743.

Maki, Y, C Ura, T Yamaguchi, T Murai, M Isahai, A Kaiho, T Yamagami, S Tanaka, F Miyamae, M Sugiyama, S Awata, R Takahashi, and H Yamaguchi. 2012. "Effects of intervention using a community-based walking program for prevention of mental decline: A randomized controlled trial." *Journal of the American Geriatrics Society* 60 (3):505-510.

Marín-Cascales, Elena, Pedro E Alcaraz, Domingo J Ramos-Campo, and Jacobo A Rubio-Arias. 2018. "Effects of multicomponent training on lean and bone mass in postmenopausal and older women: a systematic review." *Menopause* 25 (3):346-356.

Marín-Cascales, Elena, Pedro E Alcaraz, and Jacobo A Rubio-Arias. 2017. "Effects of 24 weeks of whole body vibration versus multicomponent training on muscle strength and body composition in postmenopausal women: a randomized controlled trial." *Rejuvenation research* 20 (3):193-201.

Marques, Elisa, J Carvalho, JMC Soares, F Marques, and J Mota. 2009. "Effects of resistance and multicomponent exercise on lipid profiles of older women." *Maturitas* 63 (1):84-88.

Marques, Elisa, Jorge Mota, Leandro Machado, Filipa Sousa, Margarida Coelho, Pedro Moreira, and Joana Carvalho. 2011. "Multicomponent training program with weight-bearing exercises elicits favorable bone density, muscle strength, and balance adaptations in older women." *Calcified tissue international* 88 (2):117-129.

Martínez-Amat, Antonio, Fidel Hita-Contreras, Rafael Lomas-Vega, Isabel Caballero-Martínez, Pablo J Alvarez, and Emilio Martínez-López. 2013. "Effects of 12-week proprioception training program on postural stability, gait, and balance in older adults: a controlled clinical trial." *The Journal of Strength and Conditioning Research* 27 (8):2180-2188.

Martyn-St James, Marrissa, and Sean Carroll. 2010. "Effects of different impact exercise modalities on bone mineral density in premenopausal women: a meta-analysis." *Journal of Bone Mineral Metabolism* 28 (3):251-267.

McKee, Gabrielle, Patricia M Kearney, and Rose Anne Kenny. 2015. "The factors associated with self-reported physical activity in older adults living in the community." *Age and Ageing* 44 (4):586-592.

Medicine, Australian New Zealand Society Geriatric. 2014. "Position statement – Exercise guidelines for older adults" *Australasian Journal on Ageing*. doi: https://doi.org/10.1111/ajag.12194.

Murtagh, Elaine M, Linda Nichols, Mohammed A Mohammed, Roger Holder, Alan M Nevill, and Marie H Murphy. 2015. "The effect of walking on risk factors for cardiovascular disease: an updated systematic review and meta-analysis of randomised control trials." *Preventive medicine* 72:34-43.

Ng, Marie, Tom Fleming, Margaret Robinson, Blake Thomson, Nicholas Graetz, Christopher Margono, Erin C Mullany, Stan Biryukov, Cristiana Abbafati, and Semaw Ferede Abera. 2014. "Global, regional, and national prevalence of overweight and obesity in children and adults during 1980–2013: a systematic analysis for the Global Burden of Disease Study 2013." *The lancet* 384 (9945):766-781.

Nogueira, Albernon Costa, Antônio Gomes de Resende Neto, José Carlos Aragão Santos, Leury Max da Silva Chaves, Luan Morais Azevêdo, Cauê V La Scala Teixeira, Gilmar Webber Senna, and Marzo Da Silva-Grigoletto. 2017. "Effects of a multicomponent training protocol on functional fitness and quality of life of physically active older women." *Motricidade* 13:86-93.

Patiño-Villena, P, J Juan-Martínez, A Domínguez-Domínguez, and E Martínez-Lacuesta. 2016. "Promoción de la actividad física en el municipio de murcia: 10 años del programa 4/40. Da el primer paso cuida tu salud." *Comunidad* 18 (3):3. ["Promotion of physical activity in the municipality of Murcia: 10 years of the 4/40 program. Take the first step, take care of your health." *Community*]

Rejeski, W Jack, Anthony P Marsh, Elizabeth Chmelo, and Jared J Rejeski. 2010. "Obesity, intentional weight loss and physical disability in older adults." *Obesity reviews* 11 (9):671-685.

Rezola-Pardo, Chloe, Ana Rodriguez-Larrad, Julen Gomez-Diaz, Garbiñe Lozano-Real, Itxaso Mugica-Errazquin, Maria Jesus Patiño, Iraia Bidaurrazaga-Letona, Jon Irazusta, and Susana María Gil. 2020. "Comparison Between Multicomponent Exercise and Walking Interventions in Long-Term Nursing Homes: A Randomized Controlled Trial." *The Gerontologist* 60 (7):1364-1373.

Rosa, Claudio, José Vilaça-Alves, Eduardo Borba Neves, Francisco José Félix Saavedra, Miriam Beatris Reckziegel, Hildegard Hedwig Pohl, and Daniela Zanini. 2017. "The effect of weekly low frequency exercise on body composition and blood pressure of elderly women." *Archivos de medicina del deporte: revista de la Federación Española de Medicina del Deporte y de la Confederación Iberoamericana de Medicina del Deporte* (177):9-14. [*Archives of sports medicine: journal of the Spanish Federation of Sports Medicine and the Ibero-American Confederation of Sports Medicine*]

Rosenberg, D, J Kerr, JF Sallis, GJ Norman, K Calfas, and K Patrick. 2012. "Promoting walking among older adults living in retirement communities." *Journal of Aging and Physical Activity* 20 (3):379-394.

Santanasto, AJ, BH Goodpaster, SB Kritchevsky, I Miljkovic, S Satterfield, AV Schwartz, SR Cummings, RM Boudreau, TB Harris, and AB Newman. 2017. "Body Composition Remodeling and Mortality: The Health Aging and Body Composition Study." *The journals of gerontology. Series A, Biological sciences and medical sciences* 72 (4):513-519. doi: 10.1093/gerona/glw163.

Strath, Scott J, Ann M Swartz, and Susan E Cashin. 2009. "Ambulatory physical activity profiles of older adults." *Journal of aging physical activity* 17 (1):46-56.

Street, SJ, JCK Wells, and AP Hills. 2015. "Windows of opportunity for physical activity in the prevention of obesity." *Obesity reviews* 16 (10):857-870.

Toraman, N Füsun, Alparslan Erman, and Evren Agyar. 2004. "Effects of multicomponent training on functional fitness in older adults." *Journal of Aging and Physical Activity* 12 (4):538-553.

Tudor-Locke, Catrine E, Cora L Craig, Yukitoshi Aoyagi, Rhonda C Bell, Karen A Croteau, Ilse De Bourdeaudhuij, Ben Ewald, Andrew W Gardner, Yoshiro Hatano, and Lesley D Lutes. 2011. "How many steps/day are enough? For older adults and special populations." *International journal of behavioral nutrition physical activity* 8 (1):80.

Vidarte-Claros, José Armando, Consuelo Vélez-Álvarez, Carolina Sandoval-Cuellar, and Margareth Lorena Alfonso-Mora. 2011. "Actividad física: estrategia de promoción de la salud." *Hacia la promoción de la salud* 16 (1). ["Physical activity: health promotion strategy." *Towards health promotion*]

Wang, Ray, Yuan Wang, Fang Cheng, Yuan Chao, Chien Chen, and Yea Yang. 2018. "Effects of a multicomponent exercise on dual-task performance and executive function among older adults." *International Journal of Gerontology* 12 (2):133-138.

Wareham, Nicholas J, Esther MF van Sluijs, and Ulf Ekelund. 2005. "Physical activity and obesity prevention: a review of the current evidence." *Proceedings of the Nutrition Society* 64 (2):229-247.

Watt, Jaclyn R, Jason R Franz, Keith Jackson, Jay Dicharry, Patrick O Riley, and D Casey Kerrigan. 2010. "A three-dimensional kinematic and kinetic comparison of overground and treadmill walking in healthy elderly subjects." *Clinical biomechanics* 25 (5):444-449.

WHO. 2009. *Global health risks: mortality and burden of disease attributable to selected major risks*: Geneva: World Health Organization.

INDEX

A

acromio-iliac index, 40, 59, 60, 61
adipose, 7, 10, 11, 18, 78, 79, 80, 87
adipose tissue, 7, 10, 11, 18, 78, 79, 80, 87
adiposity, x, 6, 8, 11, 17, 19, 20, 21, 75, 78, 82, 83, 84, 87, 88, 90, 110
adolescent boys, 70
adolescents, 17, 45, 53, 79, 82, 85, 88, 92, 93, 94
adults, vii, viii, ix, x, 2, 3, 6, 8, 13, 15, 17, 19, 20, 58, 76, 79, 81, 83, 85, 86, 90, 91, 92, 93, 96, 97, 98, 99, 100, 101, 102, 104, 105, 106, 107, 108, 109, 110, 111, 112, 113
adverse effects, 76
aerobic capacity, 102
aerobic exercise, 104
age, ix, 3, 5, 12, 16, 17, 40, 42, 43, 44, 45, 46, 47, 48, 49, 50, 51, 52, 53, 54, 55, 56, 57, 58, 59, 60, 61, 62, 63, 64, 65, 66, 67, 68, 69, 70, 76, 80, 83, 84, 85, 96, 101, 103
age pattern, 42, 43, 44, 48, 49, 53, 65
agricultural revolution, 69

American Heart Association, 31, 87, 93
American reference, 43, 60, 61, 70
American standards, vii, ix, 40, 43, 59, 60, 63, 67, 69
anthropometric parameter, v, vii, ix, 1, 2, 3, 5, 6, 8, 19, 21, 23, 83, 84, 92
anthropometry, 1, iii, v, vii, ix, x, 34, 39, 40, 41, 62, 65, 67, 68, 70, 71, 73, 75, 76, 78, 86, 89, 90, 92, 94, 95, 100
arm circumference (MUAC), vii, ix, 40, 41, 42, 43, 44, 51, 52, 55, 62, 63, 64, 65, 66, 79, 86, 89
assessment, x, 3, 75, 80
atherosclerosis, 9, 20, 34

B

benefits, 96, 98, 102, 103, 106, 107
biacromial breadth, ix, 40, 42, 44, 57, 58, 59, 61
biacromial ratio, 44, 62
biacromial/biiliac index, 44
biiliac breadth, ix, 40, 43, 44, 59, 60, 61
biiliac ratio, 44, 62
blood, 7, 11, 14, 84, 112

blood pressure, 7, 84, 112
body composition, vii, viii, x, 2, 5, 21, 81, 86, 89, 90, 91, 95, 96, 98, 100, 102, 103, 105, 106, 107, 109, 110, 112
body density, 80, 90
body fat, viii, x, 1, 2, 5, 12, 17, 19, 21, 75, 78, 80, 81, 82, 83, 84, 86, 87, 88, 89, 90, 92, 93, 95, 104, 105
body mass index (BMI), vii, viii, ix, x, 2, 3, 5, 7, 11, 12, 13, 14, 17, 18, 19, 21, 23, 24, 26, 30, 31, 32, 33, 35, 37, 40, 43, 44, 48, 49, 50, 62, 65, 66, 67, 68, 75, 76, 77, 78, 80, 82, 83, 84, 85, 86, 88, 89, 90, 91, 92, 93, 97
body morphology, 57, 61
body shape, 13, 58, 84
body size, 79
body surface, ix, 40, 44, 49, 50, 51, 62, 63, 64, 65
body surface area (BSA), ix, 40, 44, 49, 50, 51, 62, 63, 64, 65
body weight, 5, 8, 11, 83, 97, 100, 108
bone, x, 79, 95, 97, 98, 105, 107, 108, 109, 110, 111
bone mass, x, 95, 97, 98, 99, 105, 109, 110

C

caloric ration, 70
cardiac output, 7, 11
cardiac structure, 8
cardiovascular disease, vii, viii, ix, 2, 3, 15, 22, 23, 25, 26, 28, 29, 32, 33, 34, 35, 75, 76, 77, 80, 81, 82, 84, 85, 86, 87, 88, 92, 93, 94, 97, 98, 100, 102, 106, 107, 111
cardiovascular diseases, vii, viii, 2, 3, 77, 80
cardiovascular disorders, 3
cardiovascular function, 76, 99, 105
cardiovascular morbidity, 76, 77
cardiovascular risk, vii, ix, 2, 16, 21, 91, 92, 93

cardiovascular risk factors, v, vii, ix, 1, 2, 16, 21, 91, 92, 93
central obesity, viii, ix, 2, 6, 9, 20, 75, 76, 79, 82, 85, 94
child growth, 41, 42, 49
child mortality, 64, 65, 71
childhood, 17, 88
children, v, vii, ix, 15, 17, 27, 39, 40, 41, 42, 43, 44, 46, 48, 51, 57, 58, 59, 60, 61, 62, 64, 65, 66, 67, 68, 69, 70, 71, 73, 79, 84, 86, 88, 89, 90, 93, 111
cholesterol, 7, 10, 14, 100
chronic diseases, 16, 80
chronic obstructive pulmonary disease, 4
citizens, 98, 100, 101, 102, 103, 106
climatic changes, 68
climatic hazards, 65, 69
community, 12, 13, 72, 100, 107, 109, 110, 111
comparative advantage, 70
complex interactions, ix, 40
composition, x, 5, 88, 90, 91, 96, 105, 108
computed tomography, 18
coronary heart disease, 4, 91
cost, x, 76, 80, 82
Côte d'Ivoire, 41
crops, 68, 69

D

Dakar, 43, 69, 73
deficit, viii, ix, 40, 45, 46, 47, 48, 49, 50, 51, 52, 53, 54, 55, 56, 57, 58, 59, 61, 62, 63, 64, 66, 67, 70
Demographic and Health Surveys (DHS), ix, 40, 67, 68, 69, 71
demographic growth, 69
demographic indicator, 64
Department of Education, 95
Department of Health and Human Services, 74

developing countries, vii, viii, 1, 2, 72
DHS surveys, ix, 40, 67, 68, 69, 71
diabetes, 2, 3, 14, 15, 17, 21, 78, 83, 85, 88, 92, 100
diabetic patients, 109
diabetic retinopathy, 83, 92
diastolic blood pressure, 19
diastolic pressure, 11
diet, 9, 10, 66, 70, 89
discrimination, 15, 63
diseases, vii, 3, 15, 41, 69, 70, 91
distribution, ix, 6, 8, 21, 42, 75, 76, 77, 78, 80, 81, 83, 84, 85, 88
drought years, 65
dyslipidemia, 3, 10, 13, 16, 19, 83, 84, 105

E

economic development, viii, ix, 40, 41, 68
elderly population, 15
endurance, 99, 100, 102, 109
energy, 2, 6, 18, 70, 90, 97
environment, 53, 63, 64, 70, 98, 100, 101
environmental conditions, 98
ethnic groups, 15, 89
ethnicity, 3, 5, 78, 92
evidence, x, 3, 95, 97, 113
evolution, 55, 57, 59, 67, 68
excess body weight, 5
executive function, 102, 113
exercise program, x, 96, 99, 100, 103, 106
exercise programs, x, 96, 99, 100, 103

F

fat, ix, 2, 3, 5, 8, 12, 19, 21, 41, 42, 51, 53, 57, 66, 70, 71, 75, 76, 77, 78, 79, 80, 81, 82, 83, 87, 90, 91, 97, 98, 104
fat mass, 2, 5, 41, 42, 51, 53, 66, 70, 71, 78, 81, 90, 98
Fatick (, 65

fitness, 99, 103, 108, 111, 113
food, 2, 41, 65, 97
food aid, 65
food intake, 41
food scarcity, 65

G

gender difference, ix, 40, 70
genetic components, 76
genetic endowment, 70
growth, 6, 41, 42, 49, 69
growth factor, 6
guidelines, 88, 99, 111

H

health, vii, viii, ix, x, 1, 2, 5, 13, 14, 41, 63, 65, 72, 75, 76, 77, 78, 81, 87, 88, 96, 97, 100, 101, 102, 106, 107, 108, 110, 113
health condition, 81
health problems, 100
health risks, ix, 75, 77, 78, 87, 97, 113
height, vii, viii, ix, 2, 3, 5, 8, 13, 14, 16, 18, 19, 20, 24, 33, 34, 35, 37, 40, 41, 42, 43, 44, 46, 47, 48, 49, 51, 57, 58, 61, 62, 63, 64, 65, 66, 67, 68, 71, 78, 79, 83, 84, 85, 86, 93
hip width, 70
hips, 41, 42, 57, 59, 60, 62, 71, 78
human, vii, x, 3, 6, 75, 78, 91, 99
human body, x, 6, 75, 78, 91
hyperinsulinemia, x, 7, 75, 77
hyperlipidemia, x, 75, 77
hypertension, ix, 3, 8, 9, 12, 15, 17, 19, 75, 77, 78, 83, 85, 100
hypertriglyceridemia, 10

I

identification, 18, 82, 88, 90
iliac crest, ix, 18, 40, 43, 57, 58, 80
iliac crest height, 40, 43, 57, 58
Iliac sub-crest ratio, 44
improvements, 69, 99, 100, 103, 104, 105
individuals, viii, x, 2, 3, 5, 9, 11, 14, 21, 76, 79, 82, 83, 86, 97, 98, 102
infectious diseases, 69, 70
INSEE (Institut National des Statistiques et des Etudes Economiques), 41, 72
insulin resistance, 7
insulin sensitivity, 9

J

joint pain, 97

K

kwashiorkor, 64

L

leg length, 61, 62, 71
legs, 41, 57, 58
linoleic acid, 10
lipid metabolism, 7
lipids, 29, 70
local government, 100
local mobility, 98

M

magnitude, 48, 57, 62, 63, 65
mass, x, 2, 5, 7, 11, 12, 41, 42, 53, 66, 70, 71, 76, 78, 80, 81, 82, 83, 84, 89, 90, 91, 92, 97, 104, 105
Matam, 67

measurements, vii, ix, x, 6, 18, 21, 40, 42, 44, 65, 66, 75, 78, 80, 82, 83, 85, 86, 90, 91, 94, 96
mellitus, vii, viii, 2, 3, 78, 88
meta-analysis, 4, 5, 15, 109, 111
metabolic disorder, 89
metabolic syndrome, 2, 20, 77, 83, 87, 88, 91
minerals, 70
morbidity, 6, 14, 41, 63, 64, 79, 108
mortality, viii, ix, 2, 3, 6, 9, 12, 13, 16, 21, 22, 23, 24, 28, 30, 33, 62, 63, 64, 65, 69, 70, 71, 72, 73, 75, 76, 77, 79, 84, 87, 93, 98, 108, 112, 113
mortality risk, 16, 84
multiple regression, 14
multiple regression analysis, 14
multi-purpose survey, 41
muscle mass, x, 5, 41, 42, 51, 57, 66, 71, 95, 97, 104, 107
muscle strength, 98, 109, 110
myocardial infarction, 9, 10

N

NCHS (National Center for Health Statistics), 43, 74
NHANES (National Health and Nutrition Examination Survey), 25, 43, 74
Niakhar, ix, 40, 65, 66, 71, 73
Nigeria, 8, 25, 34
nutrition, 69, 82, 87, 88, 113
nutritional status, 44, 62, 69, 70, 71, 78, 79

O

obesity, v, vii, viii, ix, 1, 2, 3, 5, 6, 7, 9, 10, 11, 12, 13, 14, 17, 20, 21, 22, 23, 24, 25, 26, 27, 28, 29, 30, 31, 32, 33, 34, 35, 36, 37, 75, 76, 77, 78, 79, 81, 82, 83, 84, 85,

Index

86, 87, 88, 89, 90, 91, 92, 93, 94, 96, 97, 98, 106, 107, 108, 111, 112, 113
obesity prevention, 113
obstructive sleep apnea, 9, 12
overpopulated, 69
overweight, vii, viii, ix, 1, 2, 3, 5, 7, 11, 12, 14, 18, 22, 23, 27, 75, 76, 77, 79, 80, 83, 85, 86, 87, 89, 97, 111

P

participants, 4, 11, 13, 16, 17, 20, 85, 103, 104
peripheral vascular disease, 17
physical activity, 9, 11, 28, 30, 70, 82, 85, 87, 94, 96, 97, 98, 100, 101, 102, 107, 108, 109, 110, 111, 112, 113
physical exercise, viii, x, 70, 95, 96, 97, 99, 105
physical fitness, 109
physical health, 100
physical inactivity, 96
population, vii, viii, 1, 3, 13, 17, 21, 41, 42, 43, 49, 70, 72, 78, 80, 83, 84, 94, 96
population group, 96
positive correlation, 11
pre-adolescents, 45, 53
prevention, 89, 96, 99, 105, 107, 109, 110, 113
professionals, 96, 103, 106
public health, 85, 94, 96, 97, 103

Q

quality of life, 98, 102, 106, 111
quetelet index, 48

R

recovery, 55, 59, 60, 65, 98

remittances from emigrants, 69
resistance, 11, 81, 99, 104, 106, 108, 110
retarded growth, 69
risk, vii, viii, ix, 2, 3, 5, 7, 9, 10, 11, 12, 13, 14, 17, 18, 19, 20, 21, 70, 75, 76, 77, 78, 79, 80, 81, 82, 83, 84, 85, 86, 87, 88, 91, 92, 93, 94, 96, 97, 98, 102, 105, 106, 107, 108, 109, 111
risk factors, ix, 3, 9, 10, 11, 14, 18, 21, 75, 83, 85, 92, 96, 98, 108, 109, 111
rural areas, vii, ix, 40, 42, 43, 45, 48, 52, 53, 54, 57, 63, 64, 67, 70
rural population, 63

S

Sahelian, 58, 65, 71, 73
Saint-Louis, 67
sample size, 42
sarcopenia, 97, 102, 105
science, vii, x, 75, 78, 88, 92
Senegal River valley, v, vii, ix, 39, 40, 60, 65, 66, 68
sex, 3, 5, 16, 42, 43, 57, 59, 60, 63, 83
sex differences, 63, 87
shoulders, 41, 59, 60, 62
sitting height, 43
skeleton development, 41
skinfolds, ix, 40, 51, 57, 62, 63, 64, 65, 66, 70
social benefits, 102
social development, 41
social interaction, 103
social problems, 41
social support, 101
standing height, 43, 78
stature, x, 13, 43, 44, 57, 58, 59, 60, 62, 71, 75, 78, 82, 85
stunting, 46, 48, 65, 69
sub-iliac crest height, ix, 40

subscapular skinfold, ix, 40, 41, 42, 43, 54, 55, 62, 64, 66
surface area, ix, 40, 44, 49, 50, 51, 62, 63, 64, 65

T

tissue, 3, 7, 79, 80, 105, 110
tissue homeostasis, 105
traditional agriculture, 68
training, 99, 100, 102, 103, 104, 105, 106, 107, 108, 109, 110, 111, 113
training programs, 99, 103, 105
trial, 21, 106, 107, 108, 109, 110, 111
triceps, ix, 40, 41, 42, 43, 51, 53, 54, 55, 62, 63, 65, 80, 86
triceps skinfold, ix, 40, 41, 42, 43, 44, 53, 54, 55, 63, 64, 66, 86
type 2 diabetes mellitus, vii, viii, 2, 22, 78

U

under-five mortality, 62, 63, 69

urban, vii, ix, 17, 40, 41, 42, 43, 45, 47, 48, 50, 52, 53, 54, 57, 63, 64, 70, 93, 94, 100
urban areas, ix, 40, 42, 45, 47, 52, 54, 63, 70, 100
urban environment, 53, 63, 64
urban population, 17, 93

W

waist to hip ratio, vii, viii, 2, 76, 81, 82, 83, 85, 86
wasting, 48, 65
weight, vii, ix, x, 3, 4, 5, 8, 9, 11, 14, 16, 19, 20, 27, 32, 34, 40, 41, 42, 43, 44, 45, 46, 47, 48, 49, 51, 62, 63, 65, 66, 67, 68, 71, 75, 77, 78, 83, 84, 86, 93, 97, 100, 106, 108, 110, 112
weight control, 97
weight gain, 97
weight loss, 8, 97, 112
weight reduction, 9, 97